BESTSELLING BOOK SERIES

First Aid and Safety For Dummies®

Cheat Sheet

Stocking your first-aid kit

While different sources vary slightly in their opinion on what should be included, most agree on the basics.

Household items

- First-aid book
- Pencil and paper
- Change (for a phone call)
- Matches and a candle
- Blanket (those foil, "space" blankets work well and don't take up too much room)
- Tissues
- Soap
- Paper cups
- Flashlight
- Medical records
- Emergency phone numbers
- A checklist of the kit's contents

Bandages and dressings

- Adhesive bandages (assorted shapes and sizes)
- Butterfly bandages
- First-aid tape
- Elastic roller bandage (1" wide for fingers; 2" wide for wrists, hands, and feet; 3" for ankles, elbows, and arms; and 4" wide for knees and legs)
- Flexible gauze roller bandage (1" wide for fingers; 2" wide for wrists, hands, and feet; 3" for ankles, elbows, and arms; and 4" wide for knees and legs)
- Gauze pads (3" by 3" or 4" by 4")
- Eye pads
- Nonstick pads (3" by 3" or 4" by 4")
- Triangular bandage (55" across the base and 36" to 40" along each side)

First-aid equipment

- Latex gloves
- Scissors
- Tweezers
- Syringe (to squirt water and rinse out wounds)
- Thermometer
- Cotton balls
- Antiseptic wipes
- Instant cold pack
- Eye cup (to flush the eye)

Over-the-counter medications

- Antibiotic ointment (such as Neosporin)
- Antibiotic spray
- Aloe vera gel
- Ibuprofen, acetaminophen, and aspirin (**Note:** Children under the age of 21 should not take aspirin because of the risk of Reye's syndrome, a rare viral disease.)
- Topical antihistamine (such as Benadryl) or calamine lotion
- Epi-Pen (an already prepared syringe of epinephrine, available by prescription only)
- Antacid
- Motion-sickness medication (such as Bonine)
- Activated charcoal (to be used only under the direction of a poison control center)
- Syrup of ipecac (to be used only under the direction of a poison control center)
- Sterile eye wash

IDG BOOKS WORLDWIDE

Cheat Sheet $2.95 value. Item 5213-9.
For more information about IDG Books, call 1-800-762-2974.

...For Dummies®: Bestselling Book Series for Beginners

D1319171

First Aid and Safety For Dummies®

When to call, who to call

Note: This list is *only* a guide. If in doubt about a health emergency, always err on the side of caution and make the call.

Calling 911

The American College of Emergency Physicians, a group that sets standards for doctors who are specially trained to be emergency room doctors, says the following symptoms are among those serious enough to warrant a call to 911:

- Difficulty breathing or shortness of breath
- Chest or upper abdominal pain or pressure
- Fainting
- Weakness or change in vision
- Sudden, severe pain
- Bleeding that won't stop
- Severe or persistent vomiting
- Coughing up or vomiting blood
- Feelings of wanting to hurt himself or others

When you call 911, a dispatcher will ask you a series of questions. Tell the dispatcher:

- Where you're calling from
- What happened
- The age, weight, and gender of the person
- How the person is faring
- What you've done to help so far
- Any special conditions of the person (for example, pregnancy)

Calling the poison control center

If you suspect a person has ingested a poison or come in contact with a poison, contact your local poison control center. A poison is any substance that's harmful to the body, including illegal drugs, chemicals, fumes, cleaning solutions, medications, and alcohol. Poison control centers are usually open 24 hours a day, and the number for your local center can be found in the front of your phone book.

When you call the poison control center, tell the person who answers the phone:

- Who took the poison, how old he or she is, and how much the person weighs
- What the poison is (if the substance has a label, have it handy) and how much was ingested
- How the poison was taken: swallowed, inhaled, or absorbed through the skin
- What the person's condition is
- What quantity taken

Follow instructions carefully. Don't treat poisoning on your own without professional medical advice.

Calling your doctor

If you're confident a situation isn't an emergency but would still like a medical opinion, call your doctor. Most physicians have answering services that can patch you through to a doctor on call at any hour.

Praise for Family Health For Dummies

"Once or twice in a century, the paths of medical science, common sense, and clarity intersect. *Family Health For Dummies* has captured all three. A lightning strike of useful and healthy information."

—Dr. Philip P. Gerbino, President, University of the Sciences in Philadelphia

"In my lectures as president of the UCLA Center on Aging, I often say 'You can't turn the clock back — but you *can* rewind it!' That's what my friend Charles Inlander is all about in this practical guide to living *better*, longer."

—Art Linkletter, Author, Entertainer, TV Star, and President of the UCLA Center on Aging

"This book is priceless! It covers the ABCs of almost every family health question. Next to living in perfect health yourself comes the wonderful knowledge of what to do and *not* to do in any emergency. Read it before you need it!"

—Bonnie Prudden, Bonnie Prudden School and Pain Erasure Clinic

Praise for Men's Health For Dummies

"No matter how take charge they think they are, most men don't take much charge of their health. Now, thanks to Charles Inlander's *Men's Health For Dummies*, every man can take charge of his body, mind, and health. A must-read if you care at all about feeling well and staying well."

—Ted David, Network Anchor

"A smart read! Translating the newest medical discoveries into plain and fun-to-read English, Inlander tells men how to *get* healthy and how to *stay* healthy. If you want to reach your maximum potential physically and mentally, this is the resource you need."

—Sydney Walker III, M.D., Director, Southern California Neuropsychiatric Institute

"We men worry a lot about 'fitness,' but far less about what it takes for real health. Charles Inlander has boiled down tons of information to give us simple, easy-to-read rules that can make us fitter and healthier."

—Victor Cohn, former Science Editor, *The Washington Post*, Author of *News & Numbers: A Guide to Reporting Scientific Claims and Controversies in Health and Other Fields*

"Charlie cuts right to the chase. You will get the essential health information you need clearly and concisely."

—Joe Graedon, Pharmacologist, Author of the best-selling *People's Pharmacy* books

"With baby boomers aging and health costs rising, one of the most important tasks we face as a society is to persuade people to live healthier lives. This book gives men straightforward, basic advice on how to do that. I commend it to men of all ages who want to be active and healthy well into their senior years."

—Steven Findlay, Health Policy Analyst, National Coalition of Health Care

"This book is an excellent and direct approach to achieving and maintaining positive health status and possibly an excellent way to improving one's quality of life."

—J. Lyle Bootman, Ph.D., Dean and Professor, University of Arizona Health Sciences Center and Executive Director, Health Outcomes & Pharmacoeconomics Center (HOPE)

Praise for Women's Health For Dummies

"*Women's Health For Dummies* is one smart book. It's brimming with up-to-date information that all women can use to take better charge of their own health. Best of all, the book isn't patronizing or frightening. It reads instead like an invitation to better health, which is a lot harder to turn down!"

—Madge Kaplan, Health Desk Editor for public radio's night business show *Marketplace*

"*Women's Health For Dummies* helps the reader to understand — and conquer — whatever ails her. A useful guide to everything from depression to nutrition and pregnancy to breast cancer, this book helps the reader take charge of her health and her health care."

—Lori Andrews, Professor of Health Law at Chicago-Kent College of Law and Author of *The Clone Age: Adventures in the New World of Reproduction Technologies*

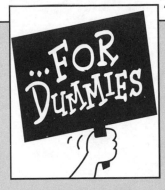

TM

References for the Rest of Us!™

BESTSELLING BOOK SERIES

Do you find that traditional reference books are overloaded with technical details and advice you'll never use? Do you postpone important life decisions because you just don't want to deal with them? Then our *...For Dummies®* business and general reference book series is for you.

...For Dummies business and general reference books are written for those frustrated and hard-working souls who know they aren't dumb, but find that the myriad of personal and business issues and the accompanying horror stories make them feel helpless. *...For Dummies* books use a lighthearted approach, a down-to-earth style, and even cartoons and humorous icons to dispel fears and build confidence. Lighthearted but not lightweight, these books are perfect survival guides to solve your everyday personal and business problems.

> *"More than a publishing phenomenon, 'Dummies' is a sign of the times."*
>
> — The New York Times

> *"A world of detailed and authoritative information is packed into them..."*
>
> — U.S. News and World Report

> *"...you won't go wrong buying them."*
>
> — Walter Mossberg, Wall Street Journal, on IDG Books' ...For Dummies books

Already, millions of satisfied readers agree. They have made *...For Dummies* the #1 introductory level computer book series and a best-selling business book series. They have written asking for more. So, if you're looking for the best and easiest way to learn about business and other general reference topics, look to *...For Dummies* to give you a helping hand.

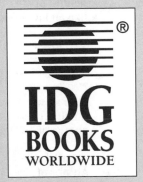

IDG BOOKS WORLDWIDE ®

1/99

First Aid & Safety

FOR DUMMIES®

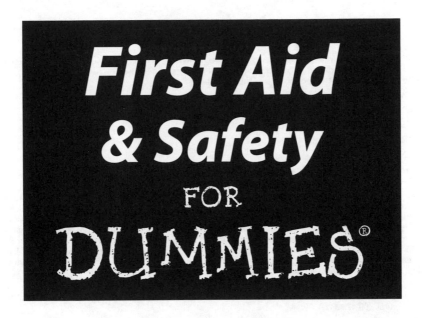

First Aid & Safety

FOR

DUMMIES®

by Charles B. Inlander, Janet Worsley Norwood, & the People's Medical Society

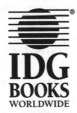

IDG Books Worldwide, Inc.
An International Data Group Company

Foster City, CA ◆ Chicago, IL ◆ Indianapolis, IN ◆ New York, NY

First Aid and Safety For Dummies®

Published by
IDG Books Worldwide, Inc.
An International Data Group Company
919 E. Hillsdale Blvd.
Suite 400
Foster City, CA 94404
www.idgbooks.com (IDG Books Worldwide Web site)
www.dummies.com (Dummies Press Web site)

Library of Congress Catalog Card No.: 99-66495

ISBN: 0-7645-5213-9

Printed in the United States of America

10 9 8 7 6 5 4 3 2 1

1B/QU/RR/ZZ/IN

Distributed in the United States by IDG Books Worldwide, Inc.

Distributed by CDG Books Canada Inc. for Canada; by Transworld Publishers Limited in the United Kingdom; by IDG Norge Books for Norway; by IDG Sweden Books for Sweden; by IDG Books Australia Publishing Corporation Pty. Ltd. for Australia and New Zealand; by TransQuest Publishers Pte Ltd. for Singapore, Malaysia, Thailand, Indonesia, and Hong Kong; by Gotop Information Inc. for Taiwan; by ICG Muse, Inc. for Japan; by Intersoft for South Africa; by Eyrolles for France; by International Thomson Publishing for Germany, Austria and Switzerland; by Distribuidora Cuspide for Argentina; by LR International for Brazil; by Galileo Libros for Chile; by Ediciones ZETA S.C.R. Ltda. for Peru; by WS Computer Publishing Corporation, Inc., for the Philippines; by Contemporanea de Ediciones for Venezuela; by Express Computer Distributors for the Caribbean and West Indies; by Micronesia Media Distributor, Inc. for Micronesia; by Chips Computadoras S.A. de C.V. for Mexico; by Editorial Norma de Panama S.A. for Panama; by American Bookshops for Finland.

For general information on IDG Books Worldwide's books in the U.S., please call our Consumer Customer Service department at 800-762-2974. For reseller information, including discounts and premium sales, please call our Reseller Customer Service department at 800-434-3422.

For information on where to purchase IDG Books Worldwide's books outside the U.S., please contact our International Sales department at 317-596-5530 or fax 317-596-5692.

For consumer information on foreign language translations, please contact our Customer Service department at 1-800-434-3422, fax 317-596-5692, or e-mail rights@idgbooks.com.

For information on licensing foreign or domestic rights, please phone +1-650-655-3109.

For sales inquiries and special prices for bulk quantities, please contact our Sales department at 650-655-3200 or write to the address above.

For information on using IDG Books Worldwide's books in the classroom or for ordering examination copies, please contact our Educational Sales department at 800-434-2086 or fax 317-596-5499.

For press review copies, author interviews, or other publicity information, please contact our Public Relations department at 650-655-3000 or fax 650-655-3299.

For authorization to photocopy items for corporate, personal, or educational use, please contact Copyright Clearance Center, 222 Rosewood Drive, Danvers, MA 01923, or fax 978-750-4470.

is a registered trademark under exclusive license to IDG Books Worldwide, Inc. from International Data Group, Inc.

About the Authors

Charles B. Inlander: Charles B. Inlander, President of the People's Medical Society, is a highly acclaimed health commentator on public radio's *Marketplace*. He is a faculty lecturer at the Yale School of Medicine and writes regularly for *Nursing Economics, The New York Times, Glamour,* and *Boardroom*. Among the many books he has authored or co-authored are *Family Health For Dummies* and *Men's Health For Dummies*.

Janet Worsley Norwood: Janet Worsley Norwood is a health writer and researcher with a background in journalism. Previously an editor for the People's Medical Society, she has co-authored several books, including *Skin: Head-to-Toe Tips for Health and Beauty* and *Understanding Diabetes*.

ABOUT IDG BOOKS WORLDWIDE

Welcome to the world of IDG Books Worldwide.

IDG Books Worldwide, Inc., is a subsidiary of International Data Group, the world's largest publisher of computer-related information and the leading global provider of information services on information technology. IDG was founded more than 30 years ago by Patrick J. McGovern and now employs more than 9,000 people worldwide. IDG publishes more than 290 computer publications in over 75 countries. More than 90 million people read one or more IDG publications each month.

Launched in 1990, IDG Books Worldwide is today the #1 publisher of best-selling computer books in the United States. We are proud to have received eight awards from the Computer Press Association in recognition of editorial excellence and three from Computer Currents' First Annual Readers' Choice Awards. Our best-selling *...For Dummies®* series has more than 50 million copies in print with translations in 31 languages. IDG Books Worldwide, through a joint venture with IDG's Hi-Tech Beijing, became the first U.S. publisher to publish a computer book in the People's Republic of China. In record time, IDG Books Worldwide has become the first choice for millions of readers around the world who want to learn how to better manage their businesses.

Our mission is simple: Every one of our books is designed to bring extra value and skill-building instructions to the reader. Our books are written by experts who understand and care about our readers. The knowledge base of our editorial staff comes from years of experience in publishing, education, and journalism — experience we use to produce books to carry us into the new millennium. In short, we care about books, so we attract the best people. We devote special attention to details such as audience, interior design, use of icons, and illustrations. And because we use an efficient process of authoring, editing, and desktop publishing our books electronically, we can spend more time ensuring superior content and less time on the technicalities of making books.

You can count on our commitment to deliver high-quality books at competitive prices on topics you want to read about. At IDG Books Worldwide, we continue in the IDG tradition of delivering quality for more than 30 years. You'll find no better book on a subject than one from IDG Books Worldwide.

John Kilcullen
Chairman and CEO
IDG Books Worldwide, Inc.

Steven Berkowitz
President and Publisher
IDG Books Worldwide, Inc.

*Eighth Annual
Computer Press
Awards ≥1992*

*Ninth Annual
Computer Press
Awards ≥1993*

*Tenth Annual
Computer Press
Awards ≥1994*

*Eleventh Annual
Computer Press
Awards ≥1995*

IDG is the world's leading IT media, research and exposition company. Founded in 1964, IDG had 1997 revenues of $2.05 billion and has more than 9,000 employees worldwide. IDG offers the widest range of media options that reach IT buyers in 75 countries representing 95% of worldwide IT spending. IDG's diverse product and services portfolio spans six key areas including print publishing, online publishing, expositions and conferences, market research, education and training, and global marketing services. More than 90 million people read one or more of IDG's 290 magazines and newspapers, including IDG's leading global brands — Computerworld, PC World, Network World, Macworld and the Channel World family of publications. IDG Books Worldwide is one of the fastest-growing computer book publishers in the world, with more than 700 titles in 36 languages. The "...For Dummies®" series alone has more than 50 million copies in print. IDG offers online users the largest network of technology-specific Web sites around the world through IDG.net (http://www.idg.net), which comprises more than 225 targeted Web sites in 55 countries worldwide. International Data Corporation (IDC) is the world's largest provider of information technology data, analysis and consulting, with research centers in over 41 countries and more than 400 research analysts worldwide. IDG World Expo is a leading producer of more than 168 globally branded conferences and expositions in 35 countries including E3 (Electronic Entertainment Expo), Macworld Expo, ComNet, Windows World Expo, ICE (Internet Commerce Expo), Agenda, DEMO, and Spotlight. IDG's training subsidiary, ExecuTrain, is the world's largest computer training company, with more than 230 locations worldwide and 785 training courses. IDG Marketing Services helps industry-leading IT companies build international brand recognition by developing global integrated marketing programs via IDG's print, online and exposition products worldwide. Further information about the company can be found at www.idg.com.   1/24/99

Authors' Acknowledgments

Creating a book is a team effort. And, in this case, the team consists of many dedicated, hard-working people. We wish to personally acknowledge their contributions and offer our most sincere thanks.

First and foremost, we'd like to thank Karla Morales, vice president of editorial services and communications for the People's Medical Society. She provided her own excellent ideas and insights into the material while seamlessly bridging the gap between author and editor. It's thanks to her that this project came off without a hitch and was such a pleasure to work on.

There are others, of course, at the People's Medical Society. Mike Donio, as always, used his research talents to track down some hard-to-find materials, never batting an eye at any request. Jennifer Hay also lent her expertise to the project, reviewing and shuffling chapters to keep everything running smoothly.

At IDG, Colleen Esterline tirelessly worked to make this the best book on the subject, and thanks, too, to her knowing eye and incisive direction. Tech reviewers Jeff Hohnstreiter and Tim Spivey carefully combed the text for possible problems.

Kathryn Born also deserves recognition for her artistic talents and professionalism as she created the illustrations featured in this book.

Special thanks to IDG Books Executive Editor Tammerly Booth who conceived the project and asked us to create it. Working with her continues to be a delight.

Finally, special thanks to Sam Norwood, who contributed to the completion of this project in a million little, but important, ways.

Publisher's Acknowledgments

We're proud of this book; please register your comments through our IDG Books Worldwide Online Registration Form located at http://my2cents.dummies.com.

Some of the people who helped bring this book to market include the following:

Acquisitions, Editorial, and Media Development

Project Editor: Colleen Williams Esterline

Executive Editor: Tammerly Booth

Technical Editors: Jeffrey Hohnstreiter, James T. Spivey

Editorial Coordinator: Maureen F. Kelly

Editorial Administrator: Michelle Vukas

Editorial Assistant: Beth Parlon

Production

Project Coordinator: E. Shawn Alysworth

Layout and Graphics: Amy M. Adrian, Angela F. Hunckler, Kate Jenkins, Barry Offringa, Tracy Oliver, Jill Piscitelli, Brent Savage, Janet Seib, Jacque Schneider, Brian Torwelle, Maggie Ubertini, Dan Whetstine

Proofreaders: Laura Albert, Sally Burton, John Greenough, Marianne Santy, Rebecca Senninger

Indexer: Liz Cunningham

Special Help
Suzanne Thomas, Constance Carlisle

General and Administrative

IDG Books Worldwide, Inc.: John Kilcullen, CEO; Steven Berkowitz, President and Publisher

IDG Books Technology Publishing Group: Richard Swadley, Senior Vice President and Publisher; Walter Bruce III, Vice President and Associate Publisher; Joseph Wikert, Associate Publisher; Mary Bednarek, Branded Product Development Director; Mary Corder, Editorial Director; Barry Pruett, Publishing Manager; Michelle Baxter, Publishing Manager

IDG Books Consumer Publishing Group: Roland Elgey, Senior Vice President and Publisher; Kathleen A. Welton, Vice President and Publisher; Kevin Thornton, Acquisitions Manager; Kristin A. Cocks, Editorial Director

IDG Books Internet Publishing Group: Brenda McLaughlin, Senior Vice President and Publisher; Diane Graves Steele, Vice President and Associate Publisher; Sofia Marchant, Online Marketing Manager

IDG Books Production for Dummies Press: Debbie Stailey, Associate Director of Production; Cindy L. Phipps, Manager of Project Coordination, Production Proofreading, and Indexing; Tony Augsburger, Manager of Prepress, Reprints, and Systems; Laura Carpenter, Production Control Manager; Shelley Lea, Supervisor of Graphics and Design; Debbie J. Gates, Production Systems Specialist; Robert Springer, Supervisor of Proofreading; Kathie Schutte, Production Supervisor

Dummies Packaging and Book Design: Patty Page, Manager, Promotions Marketing

◆

The publisher would like to give special thanks to Patrick J. McGovern, without whom this book would not have been possible.

◆

Contents at a Glance

Cartoons at a Glance

By Rich Tennant

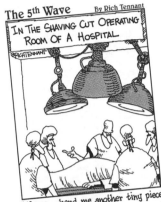

page 95

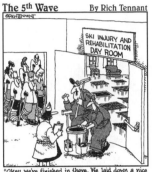

page 5

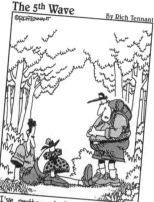

page 31

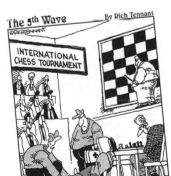

page 225

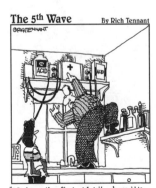

page 291

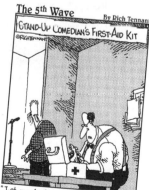

page 243

Fax: 978-546-7747 • E-mail: the5wave@tiac.net

Table of Contents

THE INFORMATION IN THIS REFERENCE IS NOT INTENDED TO
SUBSTITUTE FOR EXPERT MEDICAL ADVICE OR TREATMENT; IT IS
DESIGNED TO HELP YOU MAKE INFORMED CHOICES. BECAUSE
EACH INDIVIDUAL IS UNIQUE, A PHYSICIAN OR OTHER QUALIFIED
HEALTH CARE PRACTITIONER MUST DIAGNOSE CONDITIONS AND
SUPERVISE TREATMENTS FOR EACH INDIVIDUAL HEALTH PROB-
LEM. IF AN INDIVIDUAL IS UNDER A DOCTOR OR OTHER
QUALIFIED HEALTH CARE PRACTITIONER'S CARE AND RECEIVES
ADVICE CONTRARY TO INFORMATION PROVIDED IN THIS REFER-
ENCE, THE DOCTOR OR OTHER QUALIFIED HEALTH CARE
PRACTITIONER'S ADVICE SHOULD BE FOLLOWED, AS IT IS BASED
ON THE UNIQUE CHARACTERISTICS OF THAT INDIVIDUAL.

Introduction

In this high-tech world of ours, it's easy to overlook the basics. While most kids can surf the Web or slay a thousand evil characters on a video game, few know how to treat a wound or what to do in case of accidental poisoning. Most adults will spend the hundreds of dollars for a class on using a computer spreadsheet but pass up a free course to learn CPR.

There's no question we've let down our guard when it comes to first aid. Too many of us assume that help is always available whenever an injury or problem occurs. But the truth is too many people suffer permanent disability or die because they (or those around them) didn't know basic first aid.

But it doesn't have to be that way. First aid is not hard to learn. Knowing what to do in a medical emergency can easily mean the difference between life and death. The key is being prepared. You don't have to be a doctor, a nurse, or any other type of health professional to know basic first aid. What you need is information. And, *First Aid and Safety For Dummies* is where you'll find it.

What This Book Is About

First Aid and Safety For Dummies was written expressly for you. This is not a book for medical professionals. This is a book for the rest of us. Let's be honest about it — most of us are first-aid illiterate! Maybe you've got some emergency phone numbers hanging on the fridge. You've probably taught the little ones to wash a cut before putting on a bandage. But beyond that, if something seriously goes wrong, your first instinct is to panic.

But panicking never helped an injured person. In fact, it usually means two people are in trouble — the injured person and the panicky helper. Successful first aid starts with the person administering it — even if it's yourself — staying calm. And the best way to stay calm is by being first-aid savvy. If you know what to do and have the skills to do it, even the most serious problems can be resolved.

What sets this book apart from other first-aid guides is the approach we've taken. It's written for the whole family. It's easy to read and easy to understand. We've illustrated techniques and procedures that may be hard to figure out from words alone. Our purpose is to make first aid something anyone can do, when appropriate.

Of course, some injuries requiring first aid will require the help of a medical or EMT (Emergency Medical Technician) professional. That is clearly noted throughout the book. But, even in those situations where professional help is required, a knowledgeable layperson with first-aid knowledge can make a major difference.

Another unique aspect of the book is our focus on prevention. Knowing how to avoid a serious accident or injury is just as important — maybe more so — than knowing what to do after one occurs.

Because first aid is so important to every family, we've made sure the information and techniques found in the book are from the most knowledgeable sources. You can be confident that what you read in the following pages are what the experts say to do.

Finally, we've made sure that all the possible first aid situations you'll likely encounter are included. From sports injuries to the special needs of the elderly, disabled, and high-tech workers, it's all covered in *First Aid and Safety For Dummies.*

Foolish Assumptions

While the very nature of first aid is self-care, remember we've noted that it's not unusual to need the assistance of a medical professional under certain circumstances. Many situations requiring professional intervention are obvious. Other times it may not be so clear. That's why we say throughout the book, when in doubt call for help.

How This Book Is Organized

We've made this book easy to use by dividing it into six sections. Here's an overview of the book and what you'll find.

Part I: Let's Be Careful Out There

Knowing what to do when an emergency appears is great, but wouldn't it be better if you could head off potential problems before they arise? This part takes a look at what you can do to keep your world safer — while traveling, playing outside, or working in the home.

Part II: Be Prepared

If you're looking for the absolute basics of first aid, here's where you should start. This part gets you acquainted with the various first-aid lingo, materials, and resources. Learn when to call for help and when you can skip it. Build your own first-aid kit to suit your family's activities.

Part III: First Aid for All Occasions

This part gets into the nitty-gritty of first aid — what to do when you encounter a certain situation, such as poisoning, frostbite, heart attack, and so on. Each chapter is broken down into logical topics, such as cold exposure in one chapter and heat exposure in another. You'll also find a chapter on "sudden illnesses," those illnesses that need immediate and swift attention.

Part IV: Sports Injuries

The two chapters that make up this part present various sports and the dangers involved with them. Learn beforehand what your favorite pastime could do to your health and then customize your first-aid kit to include materials specifically needed for those injuries. It's best to be prepared!

Part V: Special Cases

Several groups of people require special care because they have special needs. This chapter introduces those groups — elderly, children, disabled persons, pregnant women, and high-tech workers. Learn prevention tips specific to these groups and see how to care for them when emergencies arise.

Part VI: The Part of Tens

Now here's a *...For Dummies* standard — the Part of Tens. This part introduces topics in a different way. The chapters offer a topic and then that topic is broken down into ten things you need to know. Look for ten ways to prepare for an emergency, ten over-the-counter products to have on-hand, ten things to know about natural remedies, and ten places to go for more information.

Icons Used in This Book

To help you get the most out of this book, we've included a few icons in the margins to point you to interesting and informative information. The following are the icons used in this book and what they mean:

This icon points to a tip that can help you make administering first aid easier.

This icon tells you to exercise caution.

This icon points to incredibly important information. Definitely read these when you run across one!

This icon tells you where we've defined some first-aid terms that would otherwise maybe trip you up.

This icon points to paragraphs specially written about children and their needs.

This icon offers alternatives to regular first-aid medications.

This icon shows you the tips and tricks of the professionals.

Where to Go from Here

You can start reading this book from cover to cover, but because we've written it so you don't have to do that, you can start anywhere and grab the information you need. You can start at the table of contents or the index to look for a specific topic. Flip to that chapter or page and you'll find the information you're looking for. We provide cross-references to other parts of the book in case you're just tuning in to that chapter and have missed some bit from earlier.

Part I
Let's Be Careful Out There

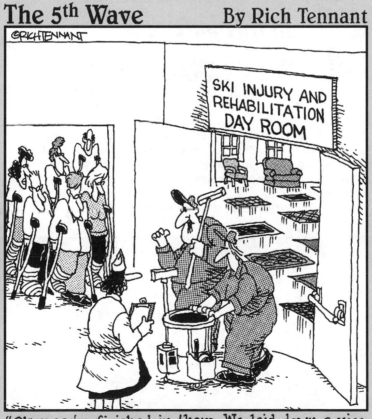

The 5th Wave   By Rich Tennant

@RICHTENNANT

SKI INJURY AND
REHABILITATION
DAY ROOM

"Okay, we're finished in there. We laid down a nice
fresh coat of wax, buffed it out real good, and then
placed some throw rugs around to spruce it up."

In this part . . .

Accidents happen, and if you worry about all the possibilities of what *could* go wrong during the course of a day, you probably wouldn't even get out of bed in the morning. But since hiding under the covers is not an option, arm yourself against emergencies with this section on prevention. You'll find information on making your home safer, avoiding basic accidents, and making decisions that decrease your risk of injury. Plus, a guide to prevention away from home steers you through the potential pitfalls of driving, biking — even walking around the block. Read this, and get ready to face the day.

Chapter 1

Making Your Environment Safe

*I*f this is a book about first aid, why, you ask, is the first section about accident prevention — something that doesn't involve first aid at all? Well, that's exactly the point. Put even a little of the information in the next two chapters to good use, and there's a good chance you can prevent some emergencies that would call for first aid. After all, first-aid skills are valuable, but they're not something you should hope you ever have to use.

In the following pages, you'll find handy hints on how to help prevent accidents in the places you live and work. The tips are arranged according to location — rooms and areas — though you'll find some suggestions can be carried over into a number of places. You'll also find discussions of fire safety, electrical safety, and clothing safety. Those of you who are eager to begin bandaging and splinting — the nitty-gritty of first aid — can skip over to Chapter 3.

The Basics of Prevention

A lot of accident prevention relies on good old common sense and some of the adages you've been hearing since you were a kid. Regardless of how many times you've heard them, they bear repeating. After all, mother knows best:

✔ Read the directions. Using an appliance or a piece of machinery in the wrong way can be dangerous, so make sure you know what you're doing before you hop on that riding mower or fire up your new food processor. Anything with moving parts should be used with caution.

- ✔ Don't run with scissors. From the halls of kindergarten come sound advice: If a child — or an adult — falls when carrying a knife, pointed stick, or other object, the result could be a nasty wound. Be careful with anything sharp — and that includes carrying sharp objects with the pointed ends facing the floor.

- ✔ Keep out of the reach of children. Common sense, for the most part, dictates what's safe for kids and what's not. Medicines, chemicals, cleaning solutions, sharp objects such as knives, tools, and toys with small parts (which may cause choking if swallowed) are just a few of the no-nos that are discussed throughout this book.

- ✔ Use the right tool for the job. Don't use a screwdriver handle to hammer home a nail. Don't scale your shelving in lieu of setting up a stepladder when replacing a hard-to-reach lightbulb. You may be asking for an accident to happen.

- ✔ Lift with your legs, not with your back. This adage may not be from childhood, but it may someday save your back. To lift correctly, stand in front of the object and plant your feet firmly. Squat down and grasp the object, keeping your back straight. Then use your thigh and leg muscles to lift the object slowly and smoothly. Lift straight up — don't twist or turn. Use the same technique when setting down an object. If you work in any job that requires lifting — such as construction or warehouse work — you'll most likely receive lessons in proper technique.

- ✔ Exercise moderation in all things. A host of health advice falls into this category. Don't drink too much, smoke, or take drugs. Watch your calorie and fat intake to stay healthy and help prevent heart disease and other conditions that may lead to an emergency situation. Don't push your body to exercise too much — or get too lazy. You can get too much of a good thing.

Safety in the Home

To help prevent accidents, you may need to move through your house, room-by-room, and make a few changes.

Kitchen

What dangers lie in the kitchen? Well, you've got a hot stove, sharp knives, bottles, and glasses — even the food itself. Here are some caveats when cooking:

✔ Stay at the stove when it's on. They say a watched pot never boils, but an unwatched pot can be a fire hazard, or cause serious burns. Turn any handles away from the front so they're not accidentally bumped, and keep children away from the hot stove. (The same holds true for the oven, which is just about at the right height for curious, exploring kids.)

✔ Make sure foods are properly cooked and stored. If you don't, food poisoning — which is especially dangerous for children and the elderly — may be the special of the day. To prevent problems, wash your hands before and after preparing food. Handle shellfish carefully, and keep sea creatures alive until you cook them. Don't get juice from raw meat on other foods, and don't baste cooked meat with marinade that held uncooked meat. Promptly put away any leftovers.

✔ When you use a knife, cut in the direction away from you — just in case the knife slips. And, of course, keep knives and scissors out of reach of children.

✔ Clean up spills on the floor right away to prevent falls.

✔ Walk carefully with hot liquids. Just a bump could send a pot of boiling water or a hot cup of tea flying.

✔ Keep appliances away from the edges of the counter so that they don't fall and injure you or a child. Also turn off appliances if you must walk away for a minute — for example, if the phone rings while you're chopping ice in a blender.

✔ Make use of smoke detectors and fire extinguishers throughout your home. The kitchen is a common scene for fire, and these two gadgets can really make a difference if one occurs. Don't limit their use to the kitchen, however — place them in appropriate spots throughout your home. Placement depends on the size and layout of your house.

✔ Use unbreakable plates and cups. If a glass or plate does break, clean it up immediately to keep tender feet from stepping on a broken shard.

Living room

Potential accidents also lurk in the living room. Here's how to keep them at bay:

✔ Make sure your fireplace is clean and covered with a screen. Don't burn anything but wood or commercial substitutes (such as those long-burning compressed wood logs) in the fireplace — other substances may burn too hot or give off dangerous fumes. Also, don't let a fire burn down unattended.

✔ Keep knickknacks away from the edges of tables and mantles. A child might knock one over or pull it down on himself.

✔ Cover your radiators. A decorative cover can help prevent burning when you brush up against a radiator. Covers, available at home improvement stores, should be properly ventilated so they don't trap heat.

✔ Don't leave lit candles unattended.

✔ Mark large windows or doors so people don't walk into them. Have you ever seen a bird fly into a window thinking it's an open door? The same thing could happen to a person.

✔ Choose carpet wisely. Select a short pile to prevent tripping, and tack down your rugs or use adhesive to secure them so they don't cause falls.

✔ Don't run electrical cords through high traffic areas or under rugs. They can trip people or get frayed and cause a fire. If you use extension cords, keep them out of the way so they're not a hazard.

Dining room

A few safety tips even come in handy during Thanksgiving dinner — or any other family meal for that matter:

✔ Cut children's food into small pieces to prevent choking. Children under age 6 shouldn't get hard candies, nuts, or big pieces of fruits or vegetables.

✔ Chew thoroughly. Although adults don't need their food cut for them, they're still at risk of choking if they're not careful. Don't rush when you eat, and try not to talk or laugh with your mouth full. Also, don't drink too much alcohol with a meal — it makes your throat lose sensation, which can contribute to choking.

✔ If you have small kids in the house, don't use a tablecloth. A little one could tug the cloth — and the silverware, glasses, plates, and candlesticks — onto the floor.

Bedroom

Want to sleep a little tighter? Here are some safety tips for the bedroom:

✔ Don't keep medicines on the bedside table. A child can easily reach them there, for one thing. Or you might reach for the wrong one (or a wrong dose) in the middle of the night.

✔ Don't smoke in bed.

✔ Use a nightlight. A little illumination may save someone — whether a kid or an adult — a fall in the middle of the night.

✔ If you have bunk beds, remember that children under 6 shouldn't be in the top bunk. Make sure the beds follow safety guidelines — check the label before you buy to see if the bed is approved, and use guardrails to keep kids in. Also, teach children not to play on or around the beds. The top bunk may seem like a perfect place to climb or jump around, but its height makes that a no-no.

✔ Use products marked *flame retardant*. While clothes and bedding cannot be made fire-proof, they can be treated to make them less likely to catch fire. Dress kids in sleepwear that is flame retardant, and look for the label on mattresses and bedspreads, too. Also be aware that different fabrics burn at different rates. Cotton burns quickly, for example, as does polyester. Polyester, however, causes especially serious burns because it melts and sticks to the skin, causing even more damage.

Bathroom

A few basic precautions can make this room much safer:

✔ Keep medications out of reach of children.

✔ Watch for slippery surfaces, like a wet tub or floor. Make sure you have skid-proof rugs or mats on all potentially slippery surfaces.

✔ Don't leave children or babies alone in the bath. A child can drown in as little as an inch of water in a matter of minutes. To make things extra safe, use a latch on the toilet seat, too. Look for them in the safety section of the toy store or in your hardware store where other childproofing supplies are found.

✔ Don't use electrical appliances near bathtubs or sinks unless they're completely dry. Even a small amount of water mixed with electricity can add up to disastrous burns or even death. The safest habit is to use your curling iron, dryer, or electric razor away from these areas entirely.

✔ Set your water heater thermostat to 120 degrees F or lower. This will help prevent scalding, which can happen quickly if tap water is too hot.

Hallways and stairways

Don't forget that accidents can happen in hallways and stairwells as well. Here are some tips to keep that from happening:

- Keep these areas free of junk such as in-line skates, tennis balls, toys, and loose papers.

- Turn on the lights when you walk down the stairs. And do just that — walk, don't run.

   To tell if your hallway or stairs are adequately lit, see if you can easily read a newspaper in the space. If you can, it's bright enough to be safe.

- Use a nightlight for dark areas.

- Make sure the railing and steps are secure.

- Mark a short flight of stairs with a bright colored carpet or plant (placed off to the side so it's not in the way) so guests and family members don't stumble.

- Make sure spindles on railings are too small for a child's head to fit through. Too wide, and they may trap a child or cause suffocation.

Garage

For many people, the garage is home to not just a car, but also a workshop, lawnmower, and a mish-mash of storage. Here's how to add safety to that mix:

- Keep pesticides and chemicals out of reach of children. Make sure all chemicals are clearly marked and in their original containers.

- At the workbench, make sure you know how to use tools before you turn them on. Follow safety guidelines provided by the manufacturer.

- Wear eye protection when you're hammering or cutting. Also wear appropriate clothing and shoes to protect against stray splinters or flying nails.

- Make sure your tools are in good working order. Store them carefully, out of the reach of children.

- Protect against the risk of fire. Keep heated tools, such as soldering irons and propane torches, safely away from greasy rags or other flammable materials. Also watch out for everyday equipment (such as a lawnmower) that may overheat and cause a fire. A good idea: Install a smoke detector and fire extinguisher.

- Keep things neat. If you open a cabinet, an avalanche of goods shouldn't tumble down onto you.

- Get sensors for your garage door opener. Safety sensors, which stop the progress of the door if an object is in the way, are now standard with most new door openers. If you have an older model, check at your hardware store on how to install them. Also make sure your door stops automatically if something interferes with the machinery.

Backyard

A little safety is in order outside of your house, too. Here are some tips:

- ✔ Don't eat plants or berries or wild mushrooms — they may be poisonous.

    This note applies especially to young children, who may be exploring the yard and taking a taste of what they find. If your kid is at this age, keep a close eye when he or she is on the prowl.

- ✔ Use insect repellent to keep stinging and biting insects away. Also watch out for snakes and spiders if they're an issue in your neighborhood.

- ✔ Stay away from strange animals. This means animals you haven't met before, as well as familiar animals that may be acting strangely. Keeping your distance will prevent bites. Plus, an animal that's walking funny or foaming at the mouth may have rabies, so keep your distance and alert local authorities if you see one.

- ✔ Wear sunscreen. Sunburn is a form of first-degree burn (or second-degree, if it involves blistering) that may require first aid.

- ✔ Take precautions if you have a pool. By law, a pool must have a locked gate, and children may not be in the pool without adult supervision. Also, don't roughhouse in a pool. If you're a pool owner, a special course in swimming and pool safety may be a good idea, and be smart and invest in lifesaving equipment such as a ring or a long pole.

- ✔ Set standards for play, and don't allow children to play unsupervised.

- ✔ Teach your kids the rules of the road. Children shouldn't play near or in the street, and they should also be taught how to properly cross a street (look both ways, cross at the corner, and so on). Bike safety precautions are also a must — more on them in Chapter 2.

- ✔ Keep bikes and toys out of the way so they don't cause falls.

- ✔ Keep kids off trampolines, even with supervision. They're dangerous.

- ✔ Use products appropriate for children. Safety standards are in place for furniture, baby supplies, toys — most things you can buy for kids — so read the label.

Fire Safety

Each year, reports the American Red Cross, some 6,000 people die in residential fires. In fact, more than 2 million such fires occur annually. Common causes include carelessness with cigarettes and matches, cooking equipment, kitchen grease, space heaters, improper storage of flammable materials, electrical problems, and malfunctioning appliances.

With those causes in mind, here are some steps you can take to keep your home safe from fire:

- ✔ Don't smoke. Aside from being bad for your health and a health hazard for those exposed to your second-hand smoke, smoking is the leading cause of fatal residential fires. If you must smoke, make sure you dispose of your cigarettes (or cigars or pipe tobacco) and matches carefully. Don't toss them out the car window (a littering offense, as well as a fire hazard) or on the ground. Instead, run water over your butts before you throw them in the wastebasket. Never throw cigarettes or ashes into a wastebasket that already contains paper. And never smoke in bed.

- ✔ Don't let kids play with matches. If you use a lighter, make sure it's child-proof — most disposable lighters have this feature.

- ✔ Have fire extinguishers and detectors in your home. Make sure smoke detectors work by checking them regularly — at least every six months. Also, once a month, look at your fire extinguisher to make sure it's full (there's a pressure gauge on the canister) and check the nozzle for obstructions or tampering.

A good time to check your smoke detector batteries is when you set the clocks ahead or behind because of daylight savings time changes in the spring and fall.

- ✔ Turn off your space heater when you're away from home or out of the room for a long period. Keep clothes and paper away from space heaters, and follow manufacturers' instructions regarding placement and proper use.

- ✔ Keep papers, potholders, and other flammable objects away from cooking surfaces in the kitchen.

- ✔ Take special care when cooking with oil or grease, because it can ignite if it gets too hot. If this occurs, smother the fire with the lid of the pot or a box of baking soda or the proper kind of fire extinguisher (see the sidebar "The ABCs (and Ds) of fire extinguishers"). *Don't* pour water on it; that will only cause the flaming oil to splash and spread.

- ✔ Watch where you use lamps, irons, toasters, and other appliances that generate heat. They reach temperatures hot enough to cause a fire.

- ✔ Don't store propane tanks (like the kind for your gas grill) in the garage. A leak can lead to a buildup of the flammable gas, and then any spark can start a blaze.

Doing the right thing when a fire strikes is also important to your safety and that of your family, so take a few minutes to review what to do.

You also need to make sure your child understands what to do if a fire occurs. While the idea of a fire might be scary for a child, they need to know what to do just as you do.

The ABCs (and Ds) of fire extinguishers

Did you know that all extinguishers aren't created equally? Different classes should be used for different things. Here are the categories and what they're used for:

✓ **Class A:** Paper, wood, trash, cloth, upholstery, rubber, and other household objects that burn easily

✓ **Class B:** Fuel, gas, grease, paint, solvents, and other flammable liquids

✓ **Class C:** Electrical equipment, such as fuse boxes and wiring

✓ **Class D:** Metals

Fortunately, you don't need to worry too much about which to choose. Most extinguishers available are approved for the A, B, and C classes. If you're working with metals, however, you may need to go the extra step.

✓ Plan an escape route for your family *before* a fire starts. Think of two ways to get out of every room in the house. Make arrangements to meet at a prearranged spot if a fire occurs so that you can see if everyone is out of the building and safe.

✓ Practice your plan. Go through the motions of evacuating the house, looking at both your ideal route and an alternate. If you're planning to climb out a window and down a trellis, make sure this is a do-able feat *before* fire actually strikes. It may not be as great an idea as you think.

✓ Get out of the building before calling for help.

✓ Don't try to rescue belongings during a fire.

✓ As you make your way out of the building, stay close to the floor. Smoke and fumes rise, and the air close to the floor will be easier to breathe.

✓ Feel a door before you open it. If it's hot to the touch, use your alternate escape route. When leaving your house, close the doors behind you. The doors will inhibit the spread of fire.

✓ If you find yourself caught in a room with a window that is too far from the ground for you to jump, open it to let in fresh air and signal rescuers by waving a cloth or sheet. Block smoke and fumes that might come in under the door with a rolled up cloth or thick rug. If possible (perhaps you're in a bathroom or utility room), make the cloth wet to increase its effectiveness.

✓ If clothing catches fire, don't run. Drop to the ground and roll around to smother the flames.

Electrical Safety

Each year in the United States, reports the Red Cross, close to 1,000 people are killed and thousands more are injured in electrical accidents. What to do for electrical burns and emergencies is described in Chapter 10. In the meantime, here are some tips for avoiding electrical accidents in the first place:

- Don't plug in, unplug, or turn off or on an appliance with wet hands. As was said before, water and electricity don't mix.

- Cover unused outlets with safety caps.

- Unplug small appliances when you're not using them. Getting into this habit will help ensure you don't leave the iron turned on or the hairdryer plugged in next to a sink of running water.

- Unplug small appliances, including your TV, computer, VCR, and stereo, during lightning storms. The wiring of your house can conduct electricity into your home if lightning strikes in the right place. For the same reason, don't use a telephone during a storm — you may get an earful of something shocking.

- Turn off the light when changing a bulb so that the socket doesn't contain live electricity. Don't use a larger watt bulb than the lamp can handle.

- Don't use extension cords for heavy duty appliances, such as a washing machine or a portable electric heater. Cords can only safely handle a certain amount of current, and too much power flowing through them may cause a fire.

- For the same reason, don't overload sockets or use too many extension cords. Not only do you create a risk of fire, the web of cords may lead to falls.

- When a fuse blows repeatedly, find out what caused the circuit to overload. Don't just flip the circuit back on or plug in a new fuse. There may be an underlying problem.

- Bind excess cords with a twist tie to keep them out of the way. This prevents wear and tear to the cords, and may also keep passersby from tripping over them.

- Check electrical appliances before use for frayed cords and other signs of wear and tear.

- Be careful with holiday lights. Make sure wires are in good repair and are being used properly. Unplug lights when they're not in use.

- Keep electrical cords out of reach of children.

Clothing and Safety

You've heard what to do about your house — your kitchen, your garage, and your backyard — plus how to keep yourself safe during a fire or when electricity is present. But there's a subject even closer to your heart (literally) than the rest of these tips: clothing.

That's right — even what you choose to wear can help prevent accidents. Here are some examples of how you can dress for success (and safety):

- ✔ Wear appropriate shoes. Proper sneakers can save your feet (and knees) if you wear them during exercise. Steel-toed boots in the workshop may keep your toes from being injured if something falls. And comfortable shoes at the office can keep you running on your feet that much longer. Overall, shoes should be comfortable and well-fitting so that you don't trip when you're wearing them or get blisters or corns from pressure.

- ✔ Wear light-colored clothing when working outside. Light colors help you find ticks (which can transmit Lyme disease) more easily.

- ✔ Wear long pants and high boots when working or walking in the brush. This keeps ticks off and protects your skin from poison ivy, brambles, and the like.

- ✔ In the summer, wear loose, light-colored clothing to prevent heat stroke.

- ✔ In the winter, dress appropriately for the cold. Put on a thermal inner layer, covered with outer garments that protect against wind and water. Cover your head and hands, and use boots and warm socks to protect your feet. Don't wear anything too tight; tight clothes prevent warm blood from circulating effectively throughout the body. Also, stay dry.

- ✔ Think in layers. Regardless of the season, give yourself some flexibility by dressing in layers of clothing. If you get too hot, just peel one off. If you're too cold, slip one on.

- ✔ Don't wear clothes with loose sleeves when cooking or using machinery. The same goes for jewelry, such as necklaces and rings. The dangling cloth or chain may catch on fire or get caught in the moving parts of the tool or appliance.

What's been presented in this chapter is simply a crash course (if you'll forgive the expression) in home safety. While the basics are covered, you can certainly do more to protect your household. For now, though, let's go on to more safety tips — this time regarding protecting yourself outside of your home, when you're on the road.

Chapter 2

Getting There Safe and Sound

• •

In This Chapter

▶ Over hill, over dale: Automobile safety

▶ Pedal power: Bicycle safety

▶ Stop, look, and listen: Pedestrian safety

▶ Off we go: Safety in the skies

▶ Have fun, but be careful: Vacation safety

▶ Too hot/too cold: Protecting against sun and frost

• •

Safety is never guaranteed, but within the walls of your home it's possible to make some changes to avoid problems *before* they start. But what do you do about safety when you venture out into the wide world? The truth is, whether you're in your car, in a plane, or on the street, you have more control than you think. The trick is knowing what to change and what to look out for.

Careful in the Car

These days, people are always on the go — to work, to the supermarket, to the kids' soccer game after school — and for most, the car is the main form of transportation. It's gotten so that we don't think twice about hopping behind the wheel, even though driving clearly has its risks. To minimize your potential for an accident, think about three important factors *before* you get into a vehicle: condition of the driver, condition of the car, and the rules of the road.

Directions for drivers

Before you drive, think about whether you *should* be driving. Keep these rules in mind:

✔ Don't drink and drive. It's not a cliché — it's lifesaving advice. Even a single drink can slow your reaction time and impair judgment, so don't be tempted to mix autos and alcohol.

✔ Don't drive if you're tired or ill. Sleepy drivers cause about 4 percent of all fatal crashes every year. If you find yourself nodding off, immediately pull over and find a safe place to sleep.

✔ Don't drive if you're taking drugs that may impair performance. Of course, this means illegal drugs, but it also means over-the-counter and prescription substances that could affect your body. A good example is antihistamines, which cause drowsiness.

About your vehicle

You wouldn't want to get on an airplane if you knew it wasn't maintained properly. But remarkably, many people climb into cars and trucks every day without knowing whether the vehicle is safe or what's beneath the hood. To reduce your risk of an accident or breakdown:

✔ Buy a "crashworthy" car. Crashworthy means the front and rear of the car absorb crashes well, keeping damage away from the driver and any passengers. What makes a car crashworthy? Four-door cars tend to be stronger than two-door cars because they have heavy steel pillars between the front and back doors. Large cars also fare better than small ones. In fact, small cars have three times the occupant death rate of bigger cars. Large cars absorb crashes better, especially when the crash is with a smaller car or moveable object. If the crash is with a fixed object, such as a tree, a larger car offers more risk of injury to the occupants because of its increased weight.

To find out if your car is crashworthy, contact the Insurance Institute for Highway Safety, an organization that evaluates cars using crash test dummies in a special testing center. The Institute's address is 1005 N. Glebe Rd., Suite 800, Arlington, VA 22201; (703) 247-1500. They're also on the Web at www.highwaysafety.org.

✔ Keep your car well serviced. Check out your lights, tires, windshield washer fluid and wipers, brakes, and steering. How often? About every six months. Also, make sure car windows, lights, mirrors, and reflectors are clean.

✔ Equip your car with safety supplies. A first-aid kit, which is described in detail in Chapter 4, should be stored along with equipment such as jumper cables, road flares, ice scraper, road atlas, rope, tool kit, matches, and a trunk tie-down — just in case!

✔ Adjust your headrest and seat belts. Your headrest, which will cushion your head during a collision, should be positioned directly behind the back of your head, and it should be locked in place. Your seat belt should be adjusted so that it's against your lap and taut against your chest and shoulder. Make sure the height is adjusted too, if your car offers that feature.

✔ Learn about airbags. Airbags have been proven to save lives. However, they've also contributed to about 113 deaths since 1993. With an impact of 20 mph, airbags are a risk to children and people of small stature who might be too close to the airbag when it is triggered by a crash.

Refinements have occurred to make airbags safer. Cars manufactured after 1998 feature airbags that inflate slower, reducing their force on passengers. Airbags are also increasingly found in the dashboard, rather than on the steering wheel, to help prevent injuries. Side airbags, which pop when your vehicle is hit from the side, help protect the chest, but they're not found in every model car — and the models that do have them tend to be pricey.

If you're a small person, give yourself at least 10 inches between the airbag cover and your chest. Slide the seat back, recline it, or move the steering wheel back a little. If you can't see the road, use a pillow to provide boost.

Kids under the age of 12 should *always* ride in the back seat. To keep babies safe, never place a rear-facing baby seat in the front seat of a car with airbags. Instead, install it in the center of the back seat or, as a second choice, in the back seat behind the passenger seat. The same goes for a convertible car seat or booster seat.

✔ Use infant and child car seats correctly. With any seat, read the owner's manual for your car and the instructions for the child safety seat. Install the seat according to the instructions so that it does not wiggle or move. Follow instructions, as well, when harnessing your child in the seat. Make sure that straps are tight and that toys and blankets don't interfere with the connection. Check that the seat is tight and the child is in correctly *each time* you go out for a drive. Connections can loosen with time.

✔ Choose an infant or child seat that meets or exceeds Federal Motor Vehicle Safety Standard 213 (check the label for this info). Don't use a hand-me-down seat if it's older than 1981, was in a crash, or shows any signs of wear and tear. Also, get a seat covered in fabric, not vinyl (which may get too hot for a baby).

Shopping for a seat?

With several different types of safety seats on the market, it pays to know which one your child will need. Here's a rundown of basic types you'll come across:

✔ **Infant seats:** These are for babies newborn to 12 months (or 16 to 22 pounds, depending on the model).

✔ **Convertible seats:** These are for newborns to 48 months.

✔ **Booster seats:** These are for kids 4 to 8 years old.

Rules of the road

If you passed your driver's test, you should know what's what when you're on the road. However, a safety-refresher doesn't hurt (though an accident might).

✔ Get everyone into seat belts. A seat belt should be worn low and tight across the lap. The shoulder strap shouldn't be close to the face (adjust the height if it is). Make sure the straps lie flat against the body, too. Impress upon your family and passengers the importance of wearing a seat belt and make it a habit they continue to live with.

✔ Stay a safe distance from the car ahead of you.

✔ Drive within the speed limit and drive defensively.

✔ Know what to do in an accident. The first thing you should do is remain calm, stop the car, and see if any injuries have occurred. If they have, call the emergency medical system (EMS) or perform first aid. You also need to get the name, address, registration, and insurance information from everyone involved in the accident — and give them your info. Don't move any car until the police arrive and direct you to do so.

✔ Know what to do in a breakdown. If your car suddenly gives out on you or suffers a flat tire, pull as far off the road as you can. Put the hood up, turn the flashers on, and set up flares behind your car. Don't put yourself at risk by going out onto the road. And unless help is definitely nearby, stay with your car.

✔ Watch out for SUVs. Sport utility vehicles give riders a high-up view of the road. That makes them more likely to flip over. Their added weight and rigidity also make them more dangerous to smaller cars they may collide with.

✔ Steer clear of drunk drivers. Even if you're sober on the road, it's likely that someone else isn't. Peak accident hours are from midnight to 3 a.m. To spot a drunk driver, watch for cars making wide turns, driving on the yellow line, weaving and swerving, following other cars too closely, or speeding and slowing down erratically.

✔ Use antilock brakes correctly. If you've been taught to pump the brakes in slippery conditions, you must change this habit if you have antilock brakes. Antilock brakes pump automatically to help your car keep its feet on slippery roads. To use them, you must put hard, continuous pressure on the pedal. You'll feel a vibration that indicates the brakes are working.

Practice stopping in slippery conditions *before* you head out on the road by stopping and starting in a deserted parking lot with puddles or light snow.

✔ Batten down the hatches. Briefcases, purses, toys, and the other stuff many people have rolling around in the car can shift or even become airborne during a sharp turn or crash. At the least, the shift may distract you from the road. At worst, a harmless object can turn into a dangerous projectile and really do some damage. Fasten stuff down before you get moving.

School bus business

If your kids catch a bus to get to class, make sure they know — and follow — these rules:

✔ Wait for the bus away from the street.

✔ Wait for the okay from the bus driver before boarding.

✔ Wear seat belts, if the bus is equipped with them.

✔ Don't fool around on the bus or distract the driver.

✔ Walk in front of the bus, never behind, when getting on or off. Stay within sight of the bus driver at all times. (Don't bend down to pick something up if it means the driver can't see you.)

Weather or not

Extreme weather — such as tornadoes, blizzards, and severe thunderstorms — may strike when you're on the road, or you may find yourself being evacuated when a hurricane or flood becomes a threat. Either way, you need to know when to stay in your car, when to leave, and how best to handle the situation.

✔ **Blizzard:** Stay in your car if you become stuck in a snowstorm, unless there's a safe place close by. As you wait, run the engine for short periods, keeping the window cracked and the exhaust pipe cleared to protect against poisoning from fumes. Put your flashes and dome lights on. Try to shift position regularly so you don't get too stiff.

✔ **Earthquake:** During an earthquake, stop your car away from buildings, trees, bridges, and overpasses. Stay in the car until the quake stops, then continue driving, avoiding bridges and underpasses (which may be damaged).

✔ **Tornado:** If you're in your car during a tornado and can't get to a sturdy building or other structure (like a highway overpass), leave the car and lie flat on the ground in a ditch with your hands over your head.

✔ **Thunderstorm:** Stay in your car. If the storm is especially fierce, pull over (away from trees or power lines) until it subsides.

✔ **Hurricane:** During hurricane season, keep a full tank of gas in your car and know the evacuation routes in your area. If you're ordered to leave, do so early. Avoid low-lying areas as you evacuate because of flooding hazards.

✔ **Flood:** Again, evacuate as soon as possible if told to do so. If you find yourself in floodwater, leave your car behind and seek higher ground. Don't drive through water — it might be deeper than you think it is.

Riding Recommendations

Bicycling is a sport and a hobby for adults and children alike. But it does come with some risks. Remember, if you're riding a bike, you're out on the road with other vehicles, following a lot of the same rules and regulations — and safety recommendations. Don't think riding a bike could be dangerous? Well, just for example, the National Center for Injury Prevention and Control reports that each year, 153,000 children get treatment in hospital emergency departments for bicycle-related head injuries.

Here's a look at what can be done:

✔ Learn the rules of the road and obey all traffic laws. Ride on the right side, with traffic — not against it. Use appropriate hand signals. Respect traffic signals. Stop at all intersections (even if they're unmarked). Look both ways before entering a street.

✔ Make sure your bike is in good working order every time you go out. Check the brakes, tires, chains, and handlebars. Also see that it's adjusted correctly to fit your height.

✔ Always wear a helmet everywhere you ride. Bicycle helmets have been shown to reduce the risk for head injury by as much as 85 percent, and the risk for brain injury by 88 percent. Says the Centers for Disease Control and Prevention, "It's a necessity, not an accessory."

✔ Wear the helmet correctly. The helmet should be snug, but comfortable. Wear it level on top of your head, not cocked backward. Use your fingers as a guide — the front of the helmet should be two fingers' width above your eyebrows. The helmet shouldn't rock when it's in place. And the straps should be buckled under your chin.

✔ Buy a helmet that meets or exceeds safety standards developed by the American National Standards Institute, the Snell Memorial Foundation, or the American Society for Testing and Materials. Check the label or ask at your sporting goods store to verify standards.

✔ Children under 10 should ride on sidewalks and paths. Before they go on the road, make sure they know the rules and have basic riding skills.

✔ Have your kids walk their bikes down the driveway. Kids riding out into the street from their own driveways is a common cause of accidents. Teach them to walk to the curb, and then look both ways before joining the flow of traffic.

✔ Don't ride at night. If visibility is poor, wear bright colors with reflective tape or other material. Make sure your bike's reflectors are clean and that you have a headlamp in good working condition.

One Step at a Time: Pedestrian Safety

If you're on foot, take care using the following tips:

✔ Cross only at intersections or marked crosswalks. Don't cross in the middle of the block.

✔ Obey traffic signals.

✔ Don't stand or cross from between two parked cars.

✔ With no sidewalk, stay on the left and walk facing traffic.

✔ Teach your children how, when, and where to cross the street.

✔ After dark or in conditions with poor visibility, carry a light or wear a highly visible outer garment, for example, one that is white or luminous.

✔ Give buses and trucks a wide berth when crossing. If you're too close to the front of the vehicle, the driver might not be able to see you.

Safety in the Skies

Yes, you do need to take precautions on planes. Plane crashes are unlikely, but they do happen. To help increase your chances of surviving during a crash, take these steps:

✔ Sit next to an exit door or close to the wings. The exit means you'll make a quicker escape, while the wing seat is protected by the plane's stronger structure.

✔ Listen to the attendant. You may have heard the spiel before, but it pays to pay attention when the flight attendant gives the preflight briefing. Be sure to take note of the closest emergency exit, and memorize the number of seats between you and it. This may help if you need to find your way out in the dark or in a smoke-filled cabin.

✔ Pick nonstop flights, if possible. Most disasters happen during takeoffs and landings.

✔ Wear your seat belt. If you're not up and moving around the cabin, keep the seat belt fastened low around your lap.

✔ Wear natural fabrics. Synthetics are more likely to ignite if there's a fire.

✔ Fly with a substantial airline. Planes with more than 30 passengers must meet strict federal safety regulations. Also look for newer planes — the lower the number (example: 737 versus 747), the older the plane is.

Vacation Situations

Away from home, at the beach, or at a campground, you'll face a whole new set of dangers and safety precautions. While you don't want to get bogged down in safety rules and regulations when you're trying to have a good time, here are some things that it won't hurt you to keep in mind:

✔ Stock up. When travelling, you want to make sure you have enough of your prescription medications to carry you through. Taking a copy of your prescription labels (and your eyeglass prescription) with you is also a good idea in case you need an emergency replacement. And don't forget about any over-the-counter products you might need, including eye care products. Tailor your travelling medicine cabinet according to need — a trip to South America will require diarrhea medication, for example.

✔ Wear sunscreen on a regular basis. Sunscreen protects against wrinkles and aging, as well as sunburn, so make it a habit to wear it every day. Look for a product marked "broad-spectrum" with a sun protection factor (SPF) of at least 15.

What does SPF indicate? It tells you how long you can be in the sun without being burned. If you usually burn within 20 minutes, for example, a product with an SPF of 15 would allow you to stay in the sun 15 times longer, or 300 minutes.

✔ Go with the shades. Just as the sun's ultraviolet rays can damage your skin, they can also harm the tissues of your eyes. To protect them, wear sunglasses that screen out broad-based UV rays. Look for a label that says "100 percent UV protection" when selecting a pair.

✔ Supervise children. Vacations are full of new places and new ways that kids can get into trouble. Keep a close eye on them at all times.

✔ Get proper instruction before you try something new or dangerous, for example, water skiing or hang gliding. Vacations are full of opportunities, but take advantage of them safely.

✔ Make sure you get enough rest and relaxation. Even though vacations are designed to let you get away from it all, you may find yourself running between destinations or attractions and wearing yourself out. So make sure to allow yourself enough time to recuperate. Otherwise, you may find yourself too tired to drive or make sound choices and decisions. You also risk injury if you play sports when you're too tired.

✔ Plan ahead. If possible, read up on medical facilities available where you're vacationing and think about where you'll go if an emergency occurs. This advice is especially apt for people travelling abroad. If you have questions, ask your travel agent for details about care in your destination.

✔ Make sure you're covered. It's a good idea to find out how your health insurance works when you're travelling and what requirements you must fulfill to receive coverage. Health maintenance organizations, especially, are fussy about covering services provided out of their regional network.

When swimming or near water

Going for a dip? Favorite vacation spots usually offer a place to take a swim, rent a boat, or even try a hand at water-skiing or parasailing. To make sure your trip is nothing but fun, think about this advice:

✔ Make sure everyone knows how to swim.

✔ Don't end up in the water unexpectedly. Stay off thin ice and away from the edge of a dock, boat, or bridge. Also steer clear of wells and cisterns. More than half of all drownings happen to people who never expected to be in the water.

✔ Know the conditions of the water. Are there riptides? Strong undercurrents? What's the depth? Also, don't trust that there's nothing down there — go into the water feet first instead of diving when in an unfamiliar place.

✔ Wear sneakers in the ocean or lakes to keep glass and critters from taking a piece of your feet.

✔ In a boat, wear a life jacket. Also, don't drink alcohol when boating. Just as you shouldn't drive a car after drinking, you shouldn't drive a boat — or even be in one, for that matter — when under the influence.

✔ Watch the weather. If you're boating, you don't want to be caught far off-shore when a storm rolls through, so keep an eye on the skies and turn back if the weather starts getting rough (and your tiny ship is tossed!). If you don't, you run the risk of capsizing or being stuck by lightening (masts tend to attract electricity). Lightening is also a risk for swimmers.

When camping

Preventing little aches and pains — and preparing for emergencies — is essential if you're heading out into the wilderness for your vacation, especially because medical help is likely to be miles and miles away. With that in mind:

✔ Don't go solo. That way, you and your companion can help each other out if necessary. Besides, you'll have someone to share your experiences with.

✔ Know where you're going. Don't leave home without a map and compass — and experience in how to use them.

✔ Fill in your friends. Telling others the specifics of your trip and where you'll be each night is a good idea. That way, if you get into trouble, others will be able to alert authorities if something's wrong and point the way for rescuers if necessary.

✔ Wear bug repellent to keep mosquitoes and other pests away.

✔ Watch out for poison ivy, poison sumac, and poison oak, which may make your trip miserable.

✔ Don't feed wild animals, for your and the animals' safety. Store food in an airtight container in your car or up in a tree — don't keep it in your tent.

✔ Check your shoes and sleeping bag before you slip in. A spider or snake might be waiting in there for you!

✔ Tell others where you're going and when you expect to be back. Don't leave without telling anyone your destination.

Temperature Time-outs

As you'll see in Chapters 16 and 17, extreme heat and cold can take their toll on your body. Heat can cause heat exhaustion, heat cramps, and heat stroke, and cold temperatures can cause frostbite and hypothermia.

To stay cool in the heat

Try these tips to help avoid heat-related illness:

- Don't overexert yourself. A strenuous workout on a hot day can earn you a heat-related illness.
- Drink plenty of water. Avoid drinks with caffeine or alcohol, which will actually speed the loss of water from your system.
- Dress in light colors and fabrics.
- Take advantage of shade and air conditioning, if it's available.
- Keep a close eye on children and the elderly. They're more susceptible to such illnesses than your average healthy adult.

To stay warm in the cold

Prevent cold temps from getting the better of you with the following advice:

- Dress in layers. Keep hands, head, and feet covered at all times. Wool is your best choice of fabric — stay away from cotton, which doesn't hold heat well.
- Don't wear clothing that is too tight. It may cut off the circulation of warm blood within your body, making you even colder.
- Move around. Exercise will keep your blood pumping.
- Drink warm liquids, but avoid caffeinated and alcoholic beverages. Caffeine and alcohol affect circulation and may make you colder.

Ideally, the precautions discussed in these first two chapters would keep any and all accidents from your doorstep. But accidents are bound to happen. The next part of this book deals with the importance of knowing first aid when an accident strikes.

Part II
Be Prepared

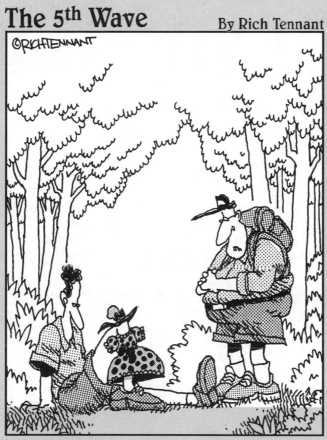

The 5th Wave — By Rich Tennant

"I've pretty much dressed the wound as well as I can, but you'll need to get to a hospital where they can more properly accessorize it."

In this part . . .

Whether you're playing sports, creating fine art, or learning first aid, the advice remains the same: Master the fundamentals. Just as a tennis player needs to have an arsenal of serves and strokes to take on an opponent, the first-aider must have a store of supplies and techniques available to thwart the effects of an accident. This part discusses those fundamentals, which include the art of stocking a first-aid kit, applying basic bandages, assessing the severity of emergencies, and rescuing victims in tough situations. First aid really starts here.

Chapter 3

First Aid: What It Is and Why You Should Know It

● ●

In This Chapter

▶ Defining first aid

▶ Understanding its importance

▶ Training for emergencies

▶ Knowing the do's and don'ts of first aid

● ●

*T*he first few chapters discuss some of the ways you can help prevent injuries when you're in your home, around your neighborhood, or on the road. Yet it's the unfortunate truth that no matter how hard you try to avoid them, accidents will happen. The best thing you can do is be prepared, and learning first aid is one of the most important ways to do just that.

What Does First Aid Mean?

Everyone knows what first aid is, right? In most people's minds, first aid means CPR, tourniquets, mouth-to-mouth resuscitation, and the MacGyver-like ability to fashion a splint out of a broken door and a shredded T-shirt. Certainly, these situations are excellent examples, but first aid can also involve much more than that.

By definition, first aid is medical care or attention provided immediately after an injury or sudden illness — before medical personnel arrive or the situation is resolved. It involves calling for help and providing lifesaving techniques, as well as more basic self-care and home remedies. It ranges from lifesaving cardiopulmonary resuscitation (CPR) to covering a child's scraped knee with an adhesive bandage decorated with smiley faces.

As you can imagine from this definition, first aid is useful in many different types of situations, ranging from a car accident with a single victim to a natural disaster, such as an earthquake, with hundreds of victims. You might use it at the ballpark during a Little League game or on a hiking trail during a camping trip. Wherever accidents and injuries can occur — and that's everywhere — first aid will come in handy.

Why Is First Aid Important?

A person with first-aid skills on the scene of an emergency can have a profound impact on the outcome of the situation. Clearly, first aid may mean the difference between life and death. But even if a situation is not life threatening, first aid is still important. Immediate care might prevent further damage that otherwise might cause permanent disability. Prompt care can also help speed healing and recovery for victims.

First aid also provides a great service to the community, especially in the event of a widespread emergency such as a natural disaster. In such situations, first aid can be used to care for many victims. Proper training can also be helpful in calming bystanders and organizing attempts at rescue.

But first aid's benefits extend beyond the victims to the rescuer. Those who know first aid have a greater sense of self-confidence and security because they know they're prepared for an unforeseen emergency. And that sense of confidence is easily transferred to victims and bystanders at the scene of an accident, making everyone involved feel more comfortable.

People well-versed in first aid can also help themselves if they're hurt or injured. Imagine you're home alone when you accidentally cut yourself badly with a paring knife. Knowing the basics of first aid may help save a trip to the emergency room.

Another benefit, of course, is the satisfaction that comes with helping a person in need — or even saving a life! But regardless of the level of care you're able to offer, first aid enables you to deal with emergency situations and know that you'll be able to do your best to help others.

Who Needs to Know First Aid?

The benefits of first aid are obvious. But honestly, how often are the Boy and Girl Scouts of the world really called upon to save lives? After all, it's not every day that you run across an accident, and with police and emergency medical technicians on call 24 hours a day, it's unlikely that a bystander would need to jump in to get the job done. Right?

Wrong. It's hard for statisticians to get a handle on how often first-aid skills are put to the test, since many instances are never reported to authorities. But these numbers should give you an idea of how common injuries are:

✔ The National Safety Council reports that at least one in four adults has suffered a nonfatal injury serious enough to need medical attention or activity restriction for at least one day.

✔ The National Center for Health Statistics (NCHS) reports that close to 94,000 deaths from accidents and unintentional injuries occurred in 1996 (the most recent year for which data were available), making accidents the fifth leading cause of death.

✔ The NCHS also reports some 43,500 motor vehicle deaths in 1996 and 4.2 million motor vehicle accident-related emergency room visits in 1995.

✔ The National Center for Injury Prevention and Control (NCIPC) reports that one teenager dies of an injury every hour of every day. In fact, injuries kill more adolescents than all diseases combined.

✔ Each year, between 20 and 25 percent of all children sustain an injury sufficiently severe to require medical attention, missed school, or bed rest, says the NCIPC.

✔ Each year, reports the NCIPC, one out of every three Americans over age 65 sustains falls.

✔ Work-related injuries accounted for 4.8 million emergency room visits in 1995, says the NCIPC.

With accidents being such common occurrences, it's easy to understand why first aid is a valuable skill for everyone to learn. But it's even more valuable for people in certain positions. Parents, for example, might learn first aid as a defense against the trouble their children could get into. And adults acting as caregivers for elderly parents might learn the ropes to ensure they can handle any health emergency they might face.

Leading causes of death in 1996

1. Heart disease	733,834	6. Pneumonia/influenza (flu)	82,579
2. Cancer	544,278	7. Diabetes	61,559
3. Stroke	160,431	8. HIV/AIDS	32,655
4. Chronic obstructive pulmonary disease	106,146	9. Suicide	30,862
5. Accidents	**93,874**	10. Chronic liver disease	25,135
		Source: National Center for Health Statistics	

Being a savvy samaritan

It seems like everyone's suing everyone else at the drop of a hat these days, which isn't reassuring to do-gooders in the world of first aid. Say you try CPR and it fails? Will the victim's family take you for all you've got? It's enough to make a person look the other way when someone's in trouble.

That's where Good Samaritan laws come in. These laws, which vary from state to state, are designed to encourage bystanders to help those in need by removing the risk of lawsuits. In a nutshell, the laws say that a person helping another person is free from liability unless he or she is grossly negligent or willfully trying to cause harm. That means you cannot be sued unless you have absolutely no idea what you're doing or are intentionally causing more pain or injury. To find out the nuances of Samaritan laws in your state, ask for information at your local library or police station, call an attorney, or talk with a local American Red Cross representative.

But first aid isn't just for the family. Teachers, for example, who routinely work with large groups of active children, should know first aid. Babysitters should know first-aid basics for their jobs. Lifeguards must know routine lifesaving techniques and first aid should an accident or injury happen on their watch. Personal trainers, coaches, and aerobics instructors also must know first aid should a sprain or strain occur. In fact, anyone who works or lives around other people — that means most of us! — should know the techniques described in these pages.

Training for First Aid

Although reading a book such as this one is a good way to learn the basics of first aid or refresh your memory regarding skills you've learned, the best way to master first aid is through a course taught by a qualified instructor. In such an atmosphere, you can see precisely how first aid is performed and you can get some practice (to some extent).

First-aid courses are offered in schools, in hospitals, at churches, and through local organizations such as the YMCA. Some companies offer first-aid training to their employees. One of the best sources for training is the American Red Cross. For information about courses they offer in your area, call your local chapter, listed in the blue pages of your telephone book. Or you can check out their Web site at www.redcross.org and enter your zip code to be directed to the chapter closest to you.

First-aid courses are often general, although many of today's programs are tailored to specific skills — for example, lifeguard training or cardiopulmonary resuscitation (CPR) training. The duration and depth of the courses vary as well, so check with the Red Cross or another source as to which program best suits your needs.

Do's and Don'ts of First Aid

Chapter 4 talks in detail about how to assess the scene of an accident or emergency and take the first steps toward care. But first, here are some general tips for first-aiders to keep in mind when they're putting their skills to good use, in the home or outside of it.

- ✔ **DO be polite:** A friend or family member will probably be comfortable with you helping them in a time of need. However, a stranger might be wary — or even afraid — of your help. An ill or injured person should be treated with respect and kindness, not treated just as a victim who needs saving. This is especially important because a person in need of aid might be shaken, scared, or in shock on account of the circumstances and therefore might be more vulnerable emotionally.

  The polite thing to do when you approach a victim you do not know is to introduce yourself — just as you would to any stranger. Find out the person's name, too, and use it as you work. Just that small bit of familiarity can calm a victim and make the situation less scary. You'll also want to mention that you've had first-aid training. After all, who wants to undergo first aid from someone who's just winging it?

  After the introductions are over, ask the person if you can help (see the item below regarding consent).

  If you need to take action that might be embarrassing to a victim (for example, removing a woman's shirt), be as sensitive as possible. Ask bystanders to move away, for example, or cover the victim with a sheet or blanket. It's a simple matter of respect.

- ✔ **DO remain calm — and calming:** Whether you're facing a situation with a friend or family member — or with a stranger — it's important to keep your wits about you and get to work. For one thing, you can't be very helpful if you're panicking. For another, taking action and, therefore, taking control of what's happening is probably the most soothing thing you can do for a victim.

  In addition, as you provide care, constantly tell the person what you're going to do and why you're doing it. Don't manhandle a victim — talk him or her through the situation. For example, you might say, "I'm going to pull up your sleeve to see how badly you've been cut" or "I'm going to roll you onto your side so you can breathe better." Explain what's going on and what will happen next. But be careful not to make any unrealistic promises — that could just make things worse.

✔ **DO obtain consent:** Once you've introduced yourself — but before you start administering first aid — you must ask and get permission from the victim to help. If a person is under age 18, you must get permission to help from his or her parents or guardian(s). This is called obtaining consent.

Consent can be refused. Although it may go against your best judgment, don't help a person who doesn't want your help. That doesn't mean you should just walk away, though. Call for help, and then stay with the victim until backup arrives.

If a person is unconscious, you'll have to assume that he or she wants your help. That's called *implied consent*. Implied consent also comes into play with children under 18 whose parents aren't available to give consent. In that circumstance, you're free to assume the parents would want you to help their child. You may also assume consent when dealing with people with mental or emotional illness who may not understand what's going on.

Sometimes it may be difficult to judge whether to proceed. To determine whether someone is alert and oriented, ask the person his or her name, date of birth, the date, and who the president is. If these questions can be answered, the person probably knows what's going on. If you're still not sure if a person who denies help is fully aware of the circumstances, it may be a good idea to let emergency medical service professionals decide—they're best equipped to evaluate the situation.

✔ **DO take precautions against infection:** Human immunodeficiency virus (HIV), the virus that causes AIDS, is a concern of health care workers today, as are a number of other infectious diseases such as herpes and hepatitis. *Remember:* Infection is also a concern of first-aid providers, who may come in contact with contaminated blood or body fluids when helping an injured person. So it's important to understand the risks.

According to the Centers for Disease Control and Prevention (CDC), there's no evidence that HIV is transmitted through saliva. And the American Heart Association reports that it does not know of any case of AIDS that resulted from mouth-to-mouth contact with a mannequin during first-aid training or from a victim of a heart attack. However, some people who perform mouth-to-mouth routinely as part of their job do use resuscitation masks, which prevent transmission of infections such as HIV and herpes.

Studies also show little risk from contact with body fluids such as urine, vomit, sweat, tears, feces, or mucus, unless they are mixed with blood.

Greater risk is associated with blood. For the most part, skin protects against infection by contaminated blood, but any small cut or sore can allow the virus an entry way into the body. The American Red Cross suggests the following to help prevent transmission:

- Avoid direct contact with blood.

- Use a clean cloth, a bandage, or latex gloves as a barrier against blood.

- Wash your hands with soap and water as soon as possible after providing first aid, whether or not you wore gloves.

- Use rubber gloves and disinfectant when cleaning up blood from surfaces. Disinfectant can be made from 1/4 cup bleach mixed with 1 gallon of water.

If you think it's likely you'll be giving first aid, you might want to think about getting a vaccination against hepatitis B, a viral illness that can be spread through contact with infected blood. Doctors call the vaccination Hep B.

✔ **DO use common sense:** It's the nature of first-aid books, including this one, to lay down the rules of what you should and shouldn't do when caring for a victim. But rules are meant to be broken, they say — at least when there's a very good reason. For example, you may know that you should never move a victim if you think he or she has a spinal cord injury. But if the car in which the victim is lying is sitting on railroad tracks with the 5:15 bearing down on it, it's in that person's best interests to pull him or her to safety. (You'll learn how in Chapter 7.)

✔ **DO stay alert:** Circumstances can change pretty quickly when there's an emergency. A fire may spread, flood waters can rise, or a building can topple. Even in less dire straits, it pays to keep an eye out for changes. That way, you can adapt and change for the best outcome.

✔ **DON'T expect too much:** True, you might have first-aid training, but that won't make you a superhero. It's possible that you'll find yourself with a victim whom you can't help. A victim might even die while you're providing aid.

That possibility shouldn't stop you from doing your best. It's important to remember that if you find that you don't have the skills to handle a particular situation, you should do what you can in other ways: Call for help, comfort the victim, and reassure the family and bystanders. If the victim can't be saved, take comfort in the fact that you did what you could.

Even so, it can be hard to deal with a traumatic circumstance — especially when you've treated victims involved. If you need some help coming to terms with a trying situation, find someone to talk with about your experience. Possibilities include a police or fire department chaplain, a member of the Salvation Army, or a counselor with experience in dealing with these types of situations.

Chapter 4

Becoming First-Aid Savvy

. . . .

In This Chapter

▶ Creating a first-aid kit

▶ Tailoring your kit for all occasions

▶ Storing and using your kit

▶ Evaluating emergencies

. . . .

*T*he carpenter wouldn't be very effective without a toolbox, and the accountant couldn't get very far without a calculator. Just as these professionals need to be equipped to handle their jobs, so must the first-aid rescuer have the right tools on hand — in the form of a first-aid kit and basic knowledge of steps to take.

Creating a First-Aid Kit

Speed is the greatest advantage of the first-aid kit: If you've prepared one ahead of time and are familiar with its contents, you have a head start when disaster strikes.

Putting together a first-aid kit is a simple task. First, grab your "toolbox," which can be anything from a cardboard box to a tote bag to a watertight case (the latter is best). The easier it is to carry, the better.

If you don't feel like going through the trouble of collecting the contents of a kit on your own, simply buy one — already complete — at the drugstore or supermarket. Sporting goods and camping supply stores also offer first-aid kits, sometimes specifically tailored to the sport or recreational activity at hand.

While different sources vary slightly in their opinion on what should be included, most agree on the basics, which include household items, such as

✔ First-aid book

✔ Pencil and paper

✔ Change (for a phone call)

- ✔ Matches and a candle
- ✔ Blanket (those foil, "space" blankets work well and don't take up too much room)
- ✔ Tissues
- ✔ Soap
- ✔ Paper cups
- ✔ Flashlight
- ✔ Medical records (see the sidebar "Maintaining medical records")
- ✔ Emergency phone numbers
- ✔ A checklist of the kit's contents

Equipment is also necessary. Stash these items in your first-aid kit:

- ✔ Latex gloves
- ✔ Scissors
- ✔ Tweezers
- ✔ Syringe (to squirt water and rinse out wounds)
- ✔ Thermometer
- ✔ Cotton balls
- ✔ Antiseptic wipes
- ✔ Instant cold pack
- ✔ Eye cup (to flush the eye)

Of course, you'll need to add bandages and dressings to your kit:

- ✔ Adhesive bandages (assorted shapes and sizes)
- ✔ Butterfly bandages
- ✔ First-aid tape
- ✔ Elastic roller bandage (1" wide for fingers; 2" wide for wrists, hands, and feet; 3" for ankles, elbows, and arms; and 4" wide for knees and legs)
- ✔ Flexible gauze roller bandage (1" wide for fingers; 2" wide for wrists, hands, and feet; 3" for ankles, elbows, and arms; and 4" wide for knees and legs)
- ✔ Gauze pads (3" by 3" or 4" by 4")
- ✔ Eye pads
- ✔ Nonstick pads (3" by 3" or 4" by 4")
- ✔ Triangular bandage (55" across the base and 36" to 40" along each side)

Maintaining medical records

An important accompaniment to a first-aid kit is the medical record. You should take the time to record pertinent medical information about each family member and keep a copy with your kit. Having details on hand can help during an emergency, when medical personnel might ask questions about medical conditions, recent care, or allergies that may affect diagnosis and treatment. Further, during a stressful situation you may not be able to focus as well, so having a medical record on hand will help you to avoid giving false information.

Include in your record the following:

✔ Emergency phone numbers (police/fire/ ambulance, poison control, doctors, and specialists)

✔ Basic health information (blood type, height, weight, blood pressure measurements, and the like)

✔ Known medical conditions

✔ Known allergies and symptoms

✔ Preventive screenings undergone and the results

✔ Immunization records for children

✔ Vision and hearing test results

✔ Hospital and laboratory records

✔ Gynecological information for women

✔ List of medications currently being taken

✔ List of conditions that may run in the family

Medications will come in handy. Add these to your first-aid kit:

✔ Antibiotic ointment (such as Neosporin)

✔ Antibiotic spray

✔ Aloe vera gel

✔ Ibuprofen, acetaminophen, and aspirin (*Note:* Children under the age of 19 should not take aspirin because of the risk of Reye's syndrome, a rare viral disease.)

✔ Topical antihistamine (such as Benadryl) or calamine lotion

✔ Epi-Pen (an already prepared syringe of epinephrine, available by prescription only)

✔ Antacid

✔ Motion-sickness medication (such as Bonine)

✔ Activated charcoal (to be used only under the direction of a poison control center)

✔ Syrup of ipecac (to be used only under the direction of a poison control center)

✔ Sterile eye wash

Wearing your info on your sleeve

If you have a particular condition, one way to pass on your medical history to emergency personnel (if you're unable to do so) is with a Medic Alert™ bracelet or pendant. The small metal tag is marked with the staff-and-serpent medical insignia on one side and your specific medical condition on the other side, along with a phone number. The phone number connects a caller with Medic Alert's emergency response center and an operator with access to your computerized medical file. The service costs $35 for the first year (which includes the standard bracelet)

and $15 for annual renewals; updates to your medical file are free. To find out more, contact Medic Alert at 800-825-3785 or see its Web site at www.medicalert.org.

Medical "smart cards" are also in development. These encoded cards, which look like credit cards, would allow medical personnel or a hospital instant access to your medical information, as well as insurance and personal info. However, their debut is still to come.

Remember to update your records regularly so that they're accurate when you need them. A good time to do this is after a doctor's appointment — the information will be fresh in your mind.

Special Circumstances, Special Kits

If someone in your life has a particular condition or if you plan to engage in a particular activity, you may want to supplement your first-aid kit with some relevant supplies.

Tailoring your kit to medical conditions

For example, if you know someone with diabetes, you should include supplies for diabetic emergencies, which include the following:

- ✔ Glucose tablets
- ✔ Disposable syringe
- ✔ Lancet (for blood sampling)
- ✔ Test strips for blood sugar
- ✔ Urine testing kit

Here's another example of circumstances in which you might consider customizing your first-aid kit. If you have a friend or family member who is severely allergic to bee stings, make sure that you have an Epi-Pen (prepared epinephrine injection) on hand. Motion-sickness medication (such as Dramamine) may come in handy if someone you know is prone to the condition.

Be sure to ask your doctor or pharmacist whether your first-aid kit is complete, based on the knowledge of your or your family members' specific medical conditions.

Taking a first-aid kit on the road

If you're preparing a kit for your car, you also want to include the following items. While not first-aid items per se, they come in handy when you're on the road.

- Flashlight
- Flares
- Nonperishable foods and water
- Electrical tape
- Fire extinguisher
- Ice scraper
- Road atlas
- Rope (about 15 feet)
- Shovel
- Jumper cables
- Tool kit
- Spare tire and jack
- Waterproof matches

Extreme heat and cold can affect medicines and supplies, and storing your first-aid kit in your car almost certainly means it will be exposed to one or the other, unless you live La-La Land where the weather is always perfect. To prevent problems, check your kit frequently to make sure its contents are complete and in good condition and discard any medications that become cloudy or discolored. If possible, remove the kit from your car when you're not using it and store it where temperatures aren't too hot or too cold.

Help is just a (cell) phone call away

If you travel frequently, you may want to invest in a cellular phone for emergencies. Having a phone on hand means that you can always call for help when needed, whether you're on a crowded highway or a deserted country road.

These days, many different types are available with a variety of calling plans. For example, you can contract with a cellular phone company for monthly service, or you can simply purchase a phone with a specific number of minutes already programmed in. Some phones are designed to make only emergency calls.

Whatever service you choose, make sure it's reliable and will operate in the regions where you travel. Also make sure your phone is always charged and in working order. Your dealer should be able to give you the details.

Preparing a kit for traveling

A first-aid and emergency kit for your own car can be as bulky as you like. But when you're traveling with only a suitcase to your name, you can't afford to pack everything from a blanket to six kinds of bandages. Here are the essentials for your times on the road.

- First-aid book
- Latex gloves
- Tweezers
- Scissors
- Thermometer
- Adhesive bandages
- Flexible gauze roller bandage
- Gauze pads
- Antibiotic ointment (such as Neosporin)
- Ibuprofen, acetaminophen, and aspirin (*Note:* Children under the age of 19 should not take aspirin because of the risk of Reye's syndrome, a rare viral disease.)
- Topical antihistamine (such as Benadryl) or calamine lotion
- Antacid
- Motion sickness medication (such as Antivert)
- Copies of prescriptions for medications currently being taken, should refills be necessary

Again, tailor your kit to the plans you're making and the places you're going. If you're headed to the beach, be sure to include sunscreen. If you're going to the desert, pack the snakebite kit. A business trip may call for mere basics, but a camping trip may be the exact opposite. Play it by ear. And follow in the footsteps of the Boy Scouts and be prepared.

Storing and Maintaining Your First-Aid Kit

Okay, you've assembled your kit. Now where do you keep it? This could be tricky because it needs to be visible and easily accessible, yet out of the reach of young children. It shouldn't be kept near heat or humidity, which makes the bathroom a far from ideal spot. Wherever you keep it, make sure that everyone in the house or workplace knows where it is. You might keep it on an eye-level shelf in the pantry, for example, or in the supply closet at the office.

It's easy to forget about a first-aid kit until you need to use it, but you should make an effort to check the contents regularly. To remind yourself, associate checking your kit with another regular task, such as replacing the batteries in your smoke detectors, resetting your clocks for daylight savings time changes, or letting your mother-in-law come for a visit.

If you use anything, be sure to replace it. Use a first-aid checklist, which should be part of your kit, and compare it with your inventory. On the same note, don't toss in items that don't belong.

Also check medications for expiration dates, and make sure bandages and equipment are up to snuff. Some medications can become discolored or cloudy or develop an odor when they're past their prime (although others may look and smell fine even though they're way past the expiration date). Even adhesive bandages can become brittle and dry when stored for too long.

Here's a brief rundown of some common medications and their shelf lives:

Cold tablets (including antihistamines)	1 to 2 years
Laxatives	2 to 3 years
Over-the-counter (OTC) painkiller tablets	1 to 4 years
Motion-sickness tablets	2 years

Go natural: An organic first-aid kit

These days, more and more people want to treat themselves and their families with natural remedies instead of medications. Well, just as you revamp your medicine cabinet to make it more natural, so can you revise your first-aid kit to achieve the same results.

To create a natural first-aid kit, start with the contents of a typical kit and make some changes. The *Natural Health First-Aid Guide* (Pocket Books, 1994) offers these natural remedies as the "top 40" for any natural kit:

✔ **Herbs:** aloe, calendula, chamomile, comfrey, echinacea, ephedra, goldenseal, ipecac, pau d'arco, plantain, slippery elm, witch hazel, and yarrow

✔ **Homeopathic remedies:** Aconite, Apis, Arnica, Arsenicum, Calendula, Hypericum, Ledum, Rhus tox, and Ruta

✔ **Flower essence:** Rescue Remedy

✔ **Essential oils:** chamomile, clove, eucalyptus, lavender, peppermint, and tea tree

✔ **Nutrition and supplements:** bromelain, papain, vitamin C, and vitamin E

✔ **Foods and household items:** activated charcoal, baking soda, cold water, garlic and onions, hydrogen peroxide, and vinegar

Warning: Part III talks about how these remedies are used, but keep in mind for now that just because a substance is characterized as natural that doesn't mean it's harmless. Some individuals may suffer allergic reactions to natural remedies, and some remedies may be dangerous if used inappropriately. In addition, remedies may also not be effective. Remember to follow instructions, and consult a medical practitioner when in doubt.

It's also smart to mark your natural first-aid kit clearly, in case anyone else might come across it. A separate, conventional first-aid kit should be kept on hand, too.

Keep in mind the difference between your first-aid kit and your medicine cabinet. Remember, the key to speed is to have a complete kit on hand at all times. Mixing your first-aid supplies into the family medicine cabinet means that you won't have what you need when you need it. On the same note, mixing unnecessary stuff in with essential first-aid equipment means you'll have to root through more — and take more time — to find what you need.

Putting Your Kit to Use

Some of the uses of items in your first-aid kit may seen apparent — for example, adhesive bandages and scissors. But the purpose of others, such as butterfly bandages, aloe vera gel, or activated charcoal, may seem more mysterious.

Don't worry, explanations can be found in Part III, in the discussions that accompany specific emergencies and how they're treated with first aid. For now, these items are just listed so that you'll have them on hand should you need them.

Evaluating Emergencies

Every first-aid situation is different, and as such, you should handle each one differently. But as you approach the scene of an accident or injury, you should follow a few basic steps that are common to most situations: In short, find out what's going on and begin to give care.

Granted, not every first-aid situation will call for the following steps. If something minor occurs — a friend slices a finger working on a wood shop project or a child trips and falls — you don't need to worry about calling for help right away or performing lifesaving measures. But in more serious situations, where every second counts, the step-by-step approach will help you make the right decisions.

The basics to begin with

The basics include the following:

- **Call for help:** Your first action in any emergency should be to call for emergency medical personnel or to send someone else to do it for you. In most communities, you can do this by calling 9-1-1. (See Chapter 6 for more on this issue, including when and when not to call.) Be sure to keep a list of emergency phone numbers by every phone to save precious minutes in an emergency.

- **See if it's safe:** Many rescuers are injured or die each year trying to help others. You don't want to barge into the scene of an accident if danger is still present. After all, you can't help someone if you become a victim yourself. So before you act, take a few seconds to survey the scene. Don't rush in if there's a risk that you could be hurt. A quick survey may also show you the cause of the accident and give clues to the person's condition.

- **Approach the victim:** Once you've determined that the scene is safe to enter, approach the victim. No matter what the injury may be, you should first check whether the person is conscious or unconscious. To do this, touch the person gently and ask, "Are you all right?" to see if you get a response. Or introduce yourself and ask the person's name, a question that may help you determine whether the victim is confused or clear-headed.

✔ **Gather more information:** If the person is conscious, he might be able to tell you what happened and how he was injured. If the person is unconscious, the circumstances may be more difficult to discern. In either case, check for a medic alert bracelet or necklace as a clue to what's wrong. Bystanders might also be able to tell you what's happened.

✔ **Check vital signs:** Part III covers taking care of specific injuries and accidents. In any situation, however, the first steps involve checking a person's vital signs to see if he or she is breathing and has a pulse. If breath or pulse is absent, you'll need to begin lifesaving measures (namely CPR) immediately.

If the person is conscious. . .

If a person is conscious, you can generally assume that he or she is breathing. If you haven't yet done so, introduce yourself, get the person's name, and ask for consent to administer first aid (Chapter 3 talks about this). Once consent has been obtained, you should check his or her pulse. The next step is to stop any bleeding. Then address any apparent injuries with appropriate first-aid measures (which Part III discusses).

Remember: Keep an eye on the person to make sure he or she continues to be conscious and breathing. If breathing or the heart rate stops, CPR will become necessary.

If the person is unconscious. . .

If a person is unconscious, immediately check to see if he or she is breathing and if the pulse is strong. You can assume that consent has been given in instances where the person is not conscious.

Taking a pulse

To take a pulse, place your middle and index fingers against the carotid artery in the neck. It can be found in the space between the voice box at the front of the neck and the muscle on the side of the neck. For infants, the pulse can be checked via the brachial artery in the arm. To do this, gently press two fingers on the inside of the arm, between the elbow and the shoulder.

Signs of spinal cord injuries

You might suspect a person has hurt the neck or back, but is there any way to tell? The circumstances of the accident might give you a clue; for example, a car accident or a fall is likely to yield spinal cord injuries, although they can occur in many other types of incidents as well. While only a medical professional can definitively diagnose such injuries, here are some signs that a spinal cord injury may be present:

✔ Ask the victim to move his or her toes or fingers. If they wiggle, that's a sign the spine is fine (which rhymes).

✔ Ask the victim to squeeze your hand. Again, pressure is positive.

✔ Run a key or hard object from the heel to the toes. If this motion, called the *Babinski test,* causes the big toe to curl downward, that's good news.

If the toes and fingers don't move, if the person can't squeeze your hand, or if the big toe points upward during the Babinski test, assume a spinal cord injury. That means that you shouldn't move the person unless absolutely necessary (for example, if the victim is in immediate danger).

Do not move a victim if you suspect an injured neck or back, as this can cause further damage. If there's a sign of such an injury (see the sidebar "Signs of spinal cord injuries"), leave the person in the position you found them and try to evaluate vital signs from there. If the person is wearing a motorcycle helmet, don't remove it. Taking the thing off will only disturb the spine, while leaving it on can actually help stabilize the injury.

The only exception to the "never move" rule is when the victim is in immediate danger — for example, lying in building that's about to collapse. In that case, it's worth the risk of moving the victim.

If there's no evidence of spinal injury, roll the person onto his or her back, trying to move the body as a unit (think of the way a log rolls, or how you'd play "steamroller" as a child). Once the person is lying on the back, tilt the head back so that the chin is raised. Place your face close to the victim's mouth to listen and feel for breathing, and keep an eye on the person's chest to see if it's rising and falling.

If a person is breathing, check for a pulse. If there is a pulse, turn your attention to any severe bleeding and then any other injury that calls for first aid.

If a person is not breathing, you'll need to start mouth-to-mouth resuscitation, in which you breathe air into the person's lungs. If air cannot be forced into the lungs, the airway may be blocked, meaning that first aid for choking (see Chapter 15) may be necessary.

If the person has no pulse, you should begin chest compressions, which help force blood through the body and keep tissues alive. Together, mouth-to-mouth and chest compressions are known as CPR. Chapter 19 talks in detail about how to perform CPR.

Each emergency situation is different. Still, the preceding steps provide the foundation for first-aid procedures and ensure that basic lifesaving measures are begun as soon as possible — regardless of why they're needed. Turn to Part III to find out how to handle specific conditions.

Learn your lifesaving letters

First-aid groups often use acronyms to describe lifesaving steps used in first aid, and their inventions may help you remember the steps.

For the American Red Cross, the acronym is ABC, which stands for Airway, Breathing, and Circulation. The words are to remind you to check to make sure that the airway is not blocked; that the victim is breathing; and that the person's heart is beating and that he or she isn't bleeding severely.

For the National Safety Council, the acronym is ABCHs. In their materials, the letters stand for Airway, Breathing, Circulation, Hemorrhage, and spinal cord injury. This, of course, follows the same lines as what the Red Cross teaches.

Chapter 5

Dressings and Bandages

. . . .

In This Chapter

▶ Knowing what you're working with

▶ Learning the do's and don'ts

▶ Applying dressings and bandages

. . . .

*B*oy Scouts win merit bandages when they learn how to tie knots. First-aiders win skill and confidence when they learn how to apply dressings and bandages. These wrappings come in handy when caring for open wounds, burns, bone and joint injuries, and many other problems. Read on to find out more.

Dressings and Bandages: Which Is Which?

A *dressing* is a protective covering that is placed directly on an open wound. Sometimes it's called a compress. The idea of the dressing is to help stop bleeding, keep the wound clean, and absorb any blood or fluid coming from the wound. It also protects the wound from further damage and eases pain. An example of a dressing is a gauze pad. See Figure 5-1 for an example of a gauze pad and for examples of other bandages.

A *bandage,* on the other hand, is a piece of cloth or other material that keeps a dressing or a splint in place. It can be used to keep pressure on the wound, help reduce swelling, and provide support for an arm or leg that's been injured. Examples include elastic roller bandages and gauze roller bandages.

Adhesive and butterfly bandages are one-piece combinations of dressings and bandages, because they're applied directly to wounds *and* hold themselves in place. In addition, separate dressings and bandages are often used together to create combinations.

Bandages, dressings, and related items included in the first-aid kit

In Chapter 4, you'll find a complete inventory for a well-stocked first-aid kit, which includes the following bandages and pads you'll need for the techniques presented in the following pages:

- Adhesive bandages
- Butterfly bandages
- Elastic roller bandage

- First-aid tape
- Flexible gauze roller bandage
- Gauze pads
- Eye pads
- Nonstick trauma pads
- Triangular bandage

A variety of products and pads is available for specific situations. A triangular bandage, for example, is a large swath of cotton cloth that can be used in many different ways. Nonstick trauma dressings, which are designed to cover but not stick to wounds, are another example.

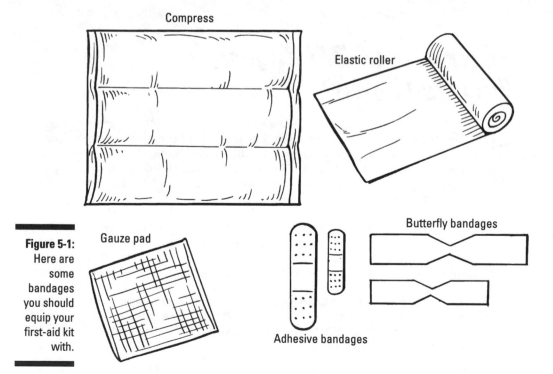

Compress

Elastic roller

Gauze pad

Butterfly bandages

Adhesive bandages

Figure 5-1: Here are some bandages you should equip your first-aid kit with.

Do's and Don'ts of Dressing

Applying a dressing or bandage is straightforward enough, but a few points should be kept in mind to avoid making matters worse. They include the following:

- ✔ **Use sterile dressings whenever possible:** *Sterile* means that the dressing is without germs, which makes sense because you don't want to expose an open wound to more germs than it already has. To keep a dressing sterile, wash your hands before handling it and don't breathe, sneeze, or cough on it. If a sterile dressing isn't available, a clean or ironed cloth can be used.

- ✔ **Apply dressings carefully so that they remain sterile:** Don't let the dressing touch any surface, including the skin of the person you're applying it to. Instead, lower it directly onto the wound. If it touches any other surface, throw it away and start over.

- ✔ **Use the right size dressing:** A dressing should extend at least 1 inch from the edge of the wound on all sides.

- ✔ **Don't use loose, fluffy cotton (such as cotton balls) on an open wound:** The material gets stuck in the wound and is hard to remove.

- ✔ **Don't remove a dressing if it gets soaked through with blood:** Just cover it with a new dressing. Dressings can be removed when bleeding stops.

- ✔ **Don't pull off a dressing that's stuck to a wound:** Let it go — pulling it off will just reopen the wound. Once bleeding has stopped completely, soak the bandage away in warm water.

Recipes for sterile dressings

Typical first-aid dressings are packaged so they remain sterile, or germ-free, until use. But you can sterilize dressings yourself in the following ways, then store them in your first-aid kit until they're needed:

- ✔ **Bake them:** Wrap a towel or cloth in aluminum foil and roast at 350 degrees F for three hours. No kidding.

- ✔ **Boil them:** Put your dressings in a pot of boiling water for 15 minutes, and then dry them where they won't become contaminated.

- ✔ **Iron them:** Not as effective as baking or boiling, ironing can be used when a dressing is needed ASAP.

It's a wrap!

Just like MacGyver could make a firecracker out of chewing gum and a piece of wire, so can you invent your own dressings and bandages should the need arise. For example, if you don't have commercial dressings, substitute a clean cloth, handkerchief, or towel. A clean sanitary napkin can stand in for a trauma dressing in a pinch. And for bandages, substitute a belt, necktie, or torn strip of cloth. Masking tape can be used in place of first-aid tape.

✔ **Be snug, not tight:** A bandage shouldn't slip off, but it shouldn't turn a person's fingers blue, either. Tingling, numbness, and a cold sensation in a limb or around the wound are symptoms that the bandage is too tight; loosen the bandage immediately if a person experiences these symptoms. Most first-aiders have trouble keeping bandages from being too loose or too tight. Use the pulse in the limb as a guideline; if you can't feel the pulse, the bandage is too tight. And be sure to check for these symptoms several times, if necessary, while waiting for help to arrive.

✔ **Let toes and fingers breathe:** To ensure good circulation when a splint is used on an arm, leg, or foot, leave the extremities exposed. Also keep an eye on them for any change in color or swelling that could indicate the bandage is too tight.

✔ **Use gauze, not elastic, roller bandages on open wounds:** Most people tend to apply the elastic too tightly. Elastic bandages are better for splints and closed injuries (injuries in which the skin is not broken or open).

✔ **Don't wrap tape all the way around:** First-aid tape can be used to secure a dressing, but winding it all the way around an arm or leg can cut off circulation, especially if swelling occurs.

Bandages for All Occasions

You might ask, what's so hard about a bandage? Isn't it basically sticking an adhesive bandage on a cut or wrapping some gauze around a wound? The truth is, there are many different types of bandages, and the kind you use depends upon what injury you're treating. In the following pages, you'll find a variety of bandaging instructions and techniques you can add to your arsenal of first-aid knowledge — which you'll rely on when you're under fire.

To tie off a bandage

You can use first-aid tape, safety pins, clips, or even masking tape to hold a bandage in place. You can also tie it off by splitting the end into two pieces, then continue wrapping one end around and tie it to the other. Yet another way is to fold the bandage back on itself, creating a loop (see Figure 5-2). Wrap the free end once more over the wound and thread it through the loop. This creates a knot.

To apply a pressure bandage

When someone is bleeding severely, a pressure bandage can help stop the flow of blood. To apply one, first elevate the wound above the level of the heart. Then place a dressing (sterile, if possible) over the wound and hold it in place with your hand (see Figure 5-3). If the dressing becomes soaked through, cover it with another one. Then place the center of the bandage over the dressing and firmly wrap both ends around the limb and tie them together. Watch for signs that the bandage is too tight, and loosen it immediately if there's any tingling or numbness or when bleeding has stopped. You can also apply pressure at one of two pressure points — the brachial artery in the arm or the femoral artery in the leg, near where it meets the pelvis — to help stop bleeding (see Figure 5-4).

Figure 5-2: Fold the bandage back on itself to create a loop. Thread the end of the bandage through the loop to create a knot.

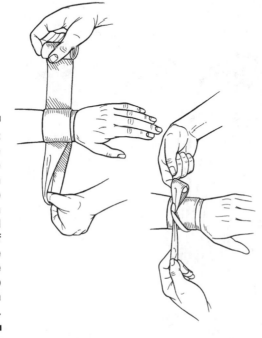

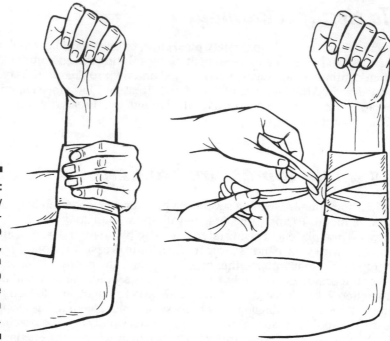

Figure 5-3:
Apply steady pressure to stop bleeding, Then use a bandage to keep the dressing in place.

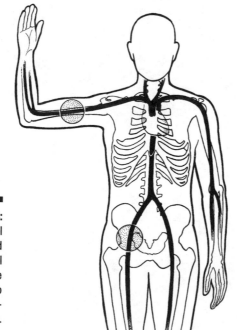

Figure 5-4:
The brachial artery and femoral artery are the two main pressure points.

To apply a tourniquet

A tourniquet is a bandage that is wrapped very tightly around a limb to stop severe bleeding or hemorrhaging. It's used in the rare instance that pressure bandages and pressure on the appropriate artery are ineffective in stopping the bleeding.

You should use tourniquets only in dire emergencies. This is because they stop the flow of blood so completely that the tissue beyond the bandage begins to die, often making amputation necessary. If you use a tourniquet, it means that you're willing to sacrifice someone's arm or leg to save his or her life. Pressure bandages do not cause tissue death unless they are wrapped too tightly.

If you decide to apply a tourniquet, note the time you put it on — you'll want to let emergency personnel know that time when they arrive on the scene. Start by placing a bandage about 2 inches wide just above the wound. Wrap it tightly around the limb two times and tie the ends together (see Figure 5-5). Then take a stick and tie it to the knot of the bandage. You should then twist the stick to further tighten the bandage — keep twisting until bleeding has stopped. Finally, keep the stick in its tightened position by tying it to the limb with another bandage. Do not remove the tourniquet from the wound once it's been applied — let emergency personnel do that job.

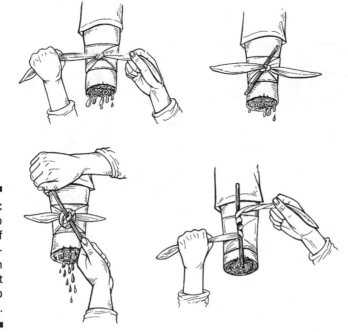

Figure 5-5:
Tie a stick to the knot of the bandage, then twist it tight to stop bleeding.

To apply a butterfly bandage

These bandages (actually a combination bandage and dressing) work best when the edges of a wound fit together — for example, in the case of a clean, sliced cut. To use one, stick one side of the adhesive bandage to one side of the wound, and then hold the wound closed as you fasten down the other side. Butterfly bandages aid healing because the edges of the wound are drawn together.

To make a ring bandage

You should use ring bandages when an object such as a pencil or knife is embedded in a wound and shouldn't be removed. To make a ring bandage, wrap a roller bandage around and around your fingers, as if you were wrapping up some loose string or ribbon (see Figure 5-6). Make the ring wide enough to fit around the embedded object. Once you have a ring of material, thread the bandage through the center of the ring and begin to wrap it around the ring itself in a spiral motion. Then fit the ring over the object and secure it with another roller bandage.

A paper cup can also be used to protect an embedded object until it can be safely removed. Simply fit the cup over the object (you may have to cut a hole in the cup's bottom if the object is taller than the cup) and fasten it in place with a roller bandage.

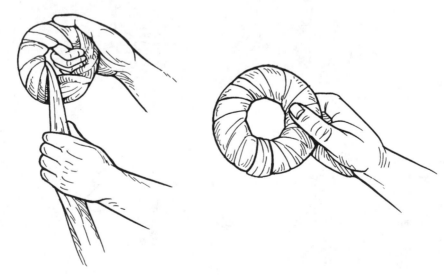

Figure 5-6:
Wrap the bandage around your fingers, then wrap it around itself to create a ring bandage.

To apply a spiral bandage

When a wound or injury is on the side of an arm and leg, a spiral bandage is used to secure a dressing in place. To apply, wrap the bandage around the limb, beginning at the bottom of the wound and working your way up in a spiral motion (see Figure 5-7). For more support, overlap the edges of the bandage. You can also wrap the bandage loosely if needed. Use a piece of first-aid tape or a safety pin to fasten the end of the bandage in place, or you can tie the bandage off.

If you need the bandage to provide more support — for example, for a large dressing or splint, use a figure-eight motion instead of a spiral, but be sure not to wrap the injury too tightly.

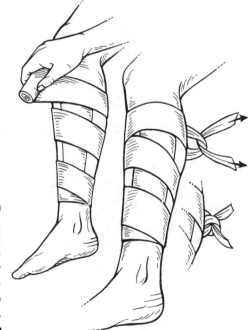

Figure 5-7:
The spiral bandage uses your basic wrap-'em-up technique.

To make an arm sling

A sling is the thing when you're dealing with a broken or wounded arm. Start with the triangular bandage from your first-aid kit: two sides should be 3 feet and the third side should be 4.5 feet. Spread the bandage over the torso of the victim, with the longest side along his or her good side and the opposite point under the elbow of the injured arm (see Figure 5-8). Take the bottom point, fold it upward over the arm, and tie it around the back of the neck to the other, topmost point. Adjust the sling so that the hand is elevated a few inches above the elbow. Pin the point at the elbow to the side of the sling to keep the arm in place. Make sure the fingers are exposed to avoid cutting off circulation.

Figure 5-8: Place the triangular bandage over the torso, under the injured arm. Fold the bottom-most point up over the arm, and tie it to the other point behind the victim's head. Fasten the corner in place.

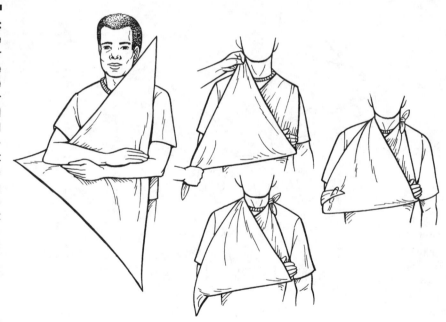

To make a cravat

To make certain types of bandages (which we describe below), you must first create a cravat. A cravat is basically your triangular bandage folded into a strip. To make one, spread the triangular bandage in front of you, with the longest side closest to you and with the point at the top (see Figure 5-9). Fold that top point toward you until it meets the center of the longest side. Then fold the top seam down again to the longest side. Keep folding until your cravat is the needed width.

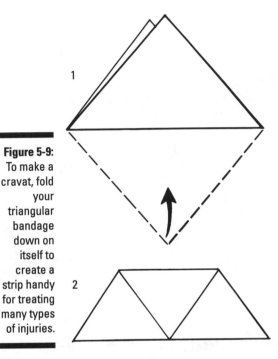

Figure 5-9:
To make a cravat, fold your triangular bandage down on itself to create a strip handy for treating many types of injuries.

To bandage the forehead or scalp

Spread your triangular bandage in front of you, with the longest side closest to you. This time, fold the bottom edge up to create a hem about 2 inches wide. Place the dressing on the wound, then lay the bandage, hem-side up, in the middle of the victim's forehead so that the point hangs toward the back of the neck (see Figure 5-10).

Next, take each side of the folded hem and wrap them around the back of the head, over the point, bringing them all the way around to the front. Tie them together. Tuck the point that's hanging down in the back over where the loop of the bandage wraps around to secure it.

Figure 5-10:
To bandage the fore-head or scalp, place the bandage on the wound with the point in the back. Then wrap both sides around the back of the head to the front and tie them together.

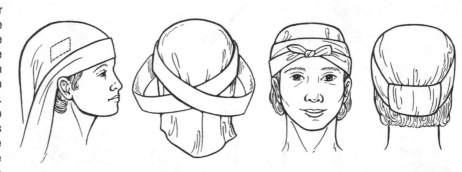

To bandage the forehead, ears, or eyes

Take your triangular bandage and make a wide cravat. Put the middle of the cravat over the dressing of the wound, and then wrap the ends around the same way you would for a head bandage (see Figure 5-11). Tie the ends again at the starting point. If you're bandaging the eyes, be sure to cover both of them. Why? Because as the uncovered, good eye moves, the injured eye will move along with it. Covering both protects against further injury.

Figure 5-11:
Place the bandage on the wound, then wrap both sides around the head to the opposite side and tie them together.

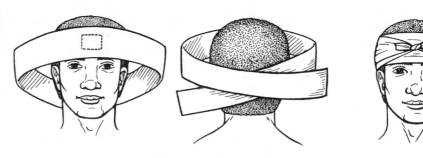

To bandage the ears or cheeks

Again, make a wide cravat and place the middle over the dressed wound. Put one end over the top of the head and the other under the chin (see Figure 5-12). At the opposite side, twist the bandage 90 degrees and continue to wrap one end around the forehead and the other end around the back of the head (think about how you wrap ribbon around a present). Tie the ends where they meet.

Figure 5-12:
Place the bandage on the wound and wrap it up and over the top of the head. Then do a 90-degree twist and wrap it around the head the other way. Tie it in place.

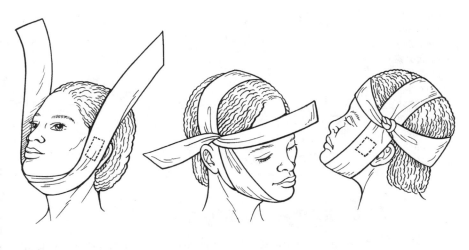

To bandage the elbow or knee

Start with the joint at a right angle and place the middle of the bandage over the dressed wound. Wrap the ends in opposite directions over and under the limb, crossing the bandage in the crook of the joint. Tie off the bandage on the side of the limb.

To bandage an ankle

To get started, place the bandage at the middle of the foot and wrap it around a few times. (see Figure 5-13). Take the bandage diagonally down around the back of the heel and back up to where you started, in a figure-eight motion. Continue this motion, overlapping each pass by about two-thirds the width of the bandage. Tie off when complete.

Figure 5-13: Wrap the bandage around the middle of the foot, then take it down around the back of the heel and back up to where you started. Use a figure-eight motion and overlap each pass as you move up and over the ankle.

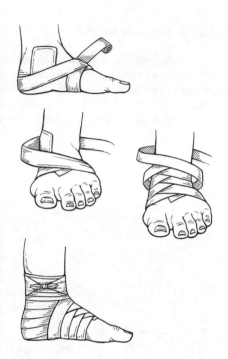

To bandage a finger

Using a narrow bandage, begin by applying the bandage vertically — up over the top of the finger and down the other side, and then doubled back on itself, up and over again (see Figure 5-14). Repeat this several times. Once the finger is wrapped vertically, hold that bandage in place with a spiral bandage wrapped horizontally and tie it off at the bottom.

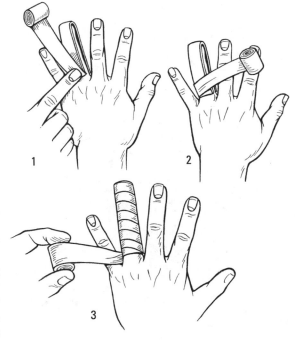

Figure 5-14:
To bandage
a finger,
wrap the
bandage
vertically
over the
injured
finger first,
then hold it
in place
with a spiral
bandage.

To bandage the hand or wrist

This bandage uses a simple figure-eight pattern. Start with the bandage over the palm, with the roll on the side away from the thumb. Wrap the bandage around the back of the hand diagonally to the wrist, just below the thumb (see Figure 5-15). Continue wrapping diagonally up over the palm, and then around the back of the hand to just above the thumb. Then cross the palm again to the opposite side of the wrist. Next, go around the back of the wrist to below the thumb and come up again into the palm. Repeat until the bandage is complete, and then tie it off.

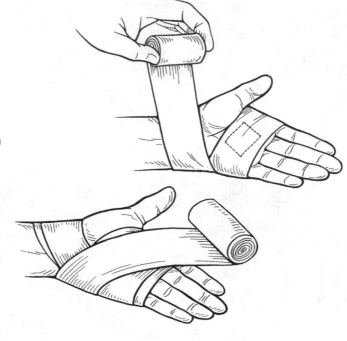

Figure 5-15:
To bandage
the hand or
wrist, wrap
the bandage
around the
palm and
the wrist
using a
figure-eight
pattern.

Where to Get Help

Getting the hang of bandages and dressings can be tough, so take some time
to practice until you get it right. (Don't practice, however, with supplies that
you plan on using in your kit — they won't be sterile when you really need to
put them in action.) A first-aid class is an excellent place to get experience.
To find one near you, contact your local chapter of the Red Cross.

Chapter 6

Who to Call and When

*F*irst aid encompasses everything from putting a bandage on a minor cut to using cardiopulmonary resuscitation (CPR) to save a life. And activating the emergency medical system (EMS) for help is one of the basics of first aid. But how can you tell whether your situation is serious enough to call professionals in for help? This chapter answers that question and offers some tips on what to expect if you do need to call.

Getting Help

In Part III, you see that the first step in providing first aid in many different types of emergencies is to go for help. In most cases, this means activating the EMS or contacting the poison control center for advice.

A list of emergency phone numbers should be placed by every phone in your home and should be inside your first-aid kit. Having those numbers on hand can save precious time in an emergency.

If you're facing an emergency alone, call for help before beginning first aid. Explain what has happened and what steps you're going to take. The exception here is if the person is not breathing or if his or her heart has stopped beating. In this situation, of course, you need to perform CPR first and foremost. Also, don't leave a person who is unconscious alone while you go for help. Stay with the person and keep an eye on vital signs.

If another person is with you, send that person for help while you begin to administer first aid. Sending two people is even better. And don't rule out sending a child for help. Today, many children are well-informed about how to call 911 in emergencies.

Kids: How they can help in a crisis

The American Medical Association says that children age 4 and above should be taught how to call for help. How do you do that? Here are some recommendations:

✔ Start by explaining to your child that he or she might need to make an important call for help someday.

✔ Teach your child how to dial 911 or another emergency number. Show your child where the number can be found next to the phone.

✔ Make sure your child knows his or her full name and complete address.

✔ Brief your child on what will happen when a call is made. Explain that a person will ask questions about the emergency and that he or she should remain calm and answer as best as he or she can.

✔ Practice making emergency calls. Using an unplugged phone, have your child dial the correct number and say his or her full name and address into the receiver.

✔ Suggest hypothetical situations to practice. For example, you might say, "What if I fell down and couldn't get up? What would you do?" Then coach your child on the correct response.

✔ Emphasize that emergency numbers should only be dialed in emergencies — never for fun!

What's EMS?

In 1973, the Emergency Medical Services Act provided for the development of integrated emergency medical systems that would serve designated geographical areas. The emergency medical system (EMS) helped train personnel (emergency medical technicians, or EMTs) establish a 911 calling system and improve communication between emergency personnel and hospital emergency rooms. It also helped categorize hospitals by their level of expertise so that EMTs could take people to the nearest hospital that would suit their needs.

Calling 911

The 911 system allows you to simply dial those three digits and immediately reach an emergency communications center. The center dispatches medical assistance instantly and may also provide help over the phone, until EMTs arrive on the scene. Some 911 centers use computer terminals that display your street address to the dispatcher automatically when you call (though this won't happen if you're on a cell phone). This is known as *enhanced 911*.

The task of developing a 911 system falls to the state, county, and municipal governments, so not every community may have a system in place. In fact, more than 50 percent of the United States is not covered by the 911 system. In some places, you can dial 911, but the call is routed to an operator who must place a call to the appropriate emergency service. In other places, dialing 0 will reach an operator who can activate the EMS.

Find out now (before there's an emergency) whether true 911 service is available in your community. If you don't have a full 911 system where you live, you may save a few valuable seconds or minutes by calling the appropriate number for your local police, fire, or ambulance service (found in the front of your phone book) and eliminating that call to the operator. You should keep that number written next to your phone so it's handy when you need it.

Should you call?

The American College of Emergency Physicians, a group that sets standards for doctors who are specially trained to be emergency room doctors, recommends that you call 911 if a person experiences

- Difficulty breathing or shortness of breath
- Chest or upper abdominal pain or pressure
- Fainting
- Weakness or change in vision
- Sudden, severe pain
- Bleeding that won't stop
- Severe or persistent vomiting
- Coughing up or vomiting blood
- Feelings of wanting to hurt himself or others

What happens when you call?

When you call 911, you'll reach a dispatcher who will ask you a series of questions. Stay on the line and calmly answer them all, beginning with where you're calling from, what happened, and how the person is faring. Also tell the dispatcher what you've done to help the victim. The information you provide will be communicated to the emergency personnel en route so that, when they arrive, they'll already have the facts and be ready to act. The 911 dispatcher may also give you instructions to follow to provide care before EMS personnel arrive.

You should post your phone number and address near every phone in your house, alongside emergency phone numbers. In an emergency, having that information in front of you may save time, especially if you're panicked or flustered. It's also important if a child or a visitor to your house (who might not know the address) needs to make an emergency call.

Calling the Poison Control Center

Local poison control centers are available throughout most of the United States to help people in emergency situations involving poisoning. The number for your local center can be found in the front of your phone book.

Poison control centers, which are open 24 hours a day in most areas of the United States, are staffed by experts who specialize in poisonings. Over the phone, they can give you first-aid instructions and information about poisonous substances. These experts are also well-informed about poisonous subjects specific to your area, because the centers are regional.

Should you call?

 If you suspect a person has ingested a poison or come in contact with a poison, contact your local poison control center. What exactly is a poison? A *poison* is any substance that's harmful to the body. Illegal drugs, chemicals, fumes, and cleaning solutions can all be poisonous, as can medications and alcohol, if used inappropriately.

What happens when you call?

When you call the poison control center, tell the person who answers the phone

- Who took the poison, how old he or she is, and how much the person weighs
- What the poison is (if the substance has a label, have it handy) and how much was ingested
- How the poison was taken: swallowed, inhaled, or absorbed through the skin
- What the person's condition is; whether he or she is unconscious or having trouble breathing; and whether he or she has a pulse
- What was the quantity taken

The poison control center expert will give you instructions to follow. For example, you may be asked to give the person activated charcoal to induce vomiting or to have the victim drink a glass of milk or water. *Follow the instructions carefully.* If detergent or gasoline has been ingested, for example, induced vomiting is not recommended.

Calling Your Doctor

Don't think that just because it's outside of office hours, you won't be able to get help from your regular doctor. Most physicians have answering services that can patch you through to a doctor on call (though maybe not your doctor) at any hour.

Should you call?

If you're confident a situation isn't an emergency but would still like a medical opinion, think about calling your doctor. However, if you're unsure whether this may be a job for emergency personnel, don't hesitate to call 911.

What happens when you call?

If it's after hours when you call your doctor's office, you most likely will reach a staffer at an answering service or hear a recording with instructions on how to contact the physician on call. Explain to the staffer that you need to speak with a doctor as soon as possible and give the details of the problem and your name and phone number. The staffer should take it from there. If you're unable to reach a physician and still feel you need medical assistance, don't hesitate to call 911.

Find out — before an emergency occurs — what your doctor's policy is on after-hours calls. He or she may have some recommendations or tips on who to contact.

When in Doubt, Call Anyway

If you're in doubt about whether a situation is an emergency, activate EMS anyway. It's better to err on the side of caution than to have a serious medical condition go untreated.

And don't worry about whether your health insurance company will make you pay for emergency room treatment because they say it wasn't a true emergency. The truth is, insurance companies rarely challenge payment for symptoms that may be life threatening. Sure, if you have a scratch or a cold, you won't be covered for ER treatment. But symptoms such as chest pain or blurry vision usually won't be questioned.

If you're in a health maintenance organization (HMO), which usually requires preapproval of care if treatments are to be covered, find out its procedure for handling medical emergencies. While HMOs don't ask you to get preapproval for emergency situations, most do require you to notify the insurance company within a certain time frame — say 24 hours — of the emergency. Make sure you know what's expected of you so that you can take the appropriate steps and ensure that you're covered. A simple call to your plan's customer service number should get your questions answered.

EMS in Action

Once you call an ambulance, who should you expect to arrive and provide care? The emergency medical system is made up of first responders, emergency medical technicians (EMTs), paramedics, and other health professionals such as doctors and nurses.

First responders are police and fire personnel who arrive on the scene before EMTs. They are trained to provide first aid and prevent further injury until EMTs arrive. If police have taken over the scene of an accident, don't interfere. Just let them do their jobs.

EMTs are specially trained personnel who staff ambulances. To become an EMT, you must complete an approved course of study comprised of 126 hours of instruction, some of it hands on. EMTs can assist in situations ranging from major trauma and serious illness to emergencies involving mental health problems. They may even defibrillate cardiac arrest patients (that is, use electricity to jump-start a stopped heart) and intubate (insert a breathing tube into) patients who've stopped breathing.

Paramedics receive more training than EMTs. They're qualified to administer medications and intravenous lines and have training in advanced life-support systems. They also use radios and other equipment to communicate with doctors and nurses in hospital emergency rooms. Not every community's EMS uses paramedics.

Finally, the team includes doctors and nurses, who take over upon arrival in the emergency room. Sometimes, they're even part of the ambulance crew, serving alongside EMTs and paramedics. Some physicians become specialists in emergency medicine, sometimes taking extra training in the field.

Off to the Emergency Room

Not all emergency rooms are created equal. While some large, well-equipped hospitals are able to handle seriously ill or injured patients, some medium-size and small hospitals don't have the resources to handle such cases.

To help patients get the care they need, the Joint Commission on the Accreditation of Healthcare Organizations (JCAHO) has categorized the capabilities of hospitals into a system of four levels of trauma care:

- **Level I:** This is the most sophisticated level of service, offering comprehensive emergency care 24 hours a day. This trauma department is staffed full-time by physicians specially trained in emergency care. Additional coverage is provided by hospital staff physicians and specialists available for consultation within 30 minutes.

- **Level II:** These emergency departments also provide comprehensive emergency care and are staffed by a least one physician who specializes in emergency medicine. Other specialists must be available for consultation within 30 minutes.

- **Level III:** These departments are available to provide care 24 hours a day. However, a physician is not necessarily physically present in the emergency room at all times, but must be available within 30 minutes of the need for care. Often, level III facilities stabilize patients before transferring them to other hospitals.

- **Level IV:** A level IV department is not much more than an aid station that can determine if an emergency exists, render first aid, and arrange for transfer of a patient to a larger facility.

The system calls for patients to be taken to the hospital best suited to their needs. Someone with very serious injuries would go to a level I hospital, for example. If that hospital were too crowded or too far away, a patient would be routed to a level II or level III facility. Likewise, a seriously ill patient who arrives at a level III facility could be transferred to a level I hospital through the system.

Getting help at an urgicenter

Emergency care is also available at *urgicenters*, those streetside clinics that are open (sometimes 24 hours a day) to walk-in patients.

Warning: Urgicenters aren't not recommended for life-threatening emergencies unless no other option is available. These centers are ideal for treating splinters, sunburns, elbow scrapes, and other minor injuries, but they're not substitutes for the high-tech care of hospital emergency departments.

Navigating the ER

On the way to the hospital, you may accompany the victim in the ambulance or be following in your own car. Once you arrive at the emergency room (ER), the injured person will be assessed by a medical professional and the case will be assigned a priority. This process is called *triage,* and it's done to make sure that serious cases are treated before minor ones. If other, more serious cases are ahead of the victim's, you may need to wait.

A medical professional will then see the victim and create a medical record for the case. The person will be asked to sign a consent form. Then, the person will be taken to an examination room for evaluation and treatment.

You may or may not be permitted to go along when a friend or family member is receiving treatment. In either instance, you should act as a patient advocate, talking with the practitioners about what's being done, providing any needed information, and explaining to the victim what's going on when you can.

Emergency room visits often end with the practitioner discharging the patient with instructions for care or a prescription. In other cases, the person may be admitted to the hospital for further treatment. Whatever the case, you can be confident that your quick alert and your first-aid skills helped get the person much needed care and attention.

Chapter 7

Emergency Rescue Procedures

● ●

In This Chapter

▶ Defining emergency rescue

▶ Knowing when rescue is necessary

▶ Moving a first-aid victim

▶ Rescuing victims in different situations

● ●

First aid means providing preliminary medical care to someone who's been hurt. But sometimes, a person needs to be taken out of harm's way even before first aid can be offered. How to rescue a wounded or injured person without causing more harm is the subject of this chapter.

Emergency Rescue: When Is It Needed?

To rescue a victim means to go in and move the person out of danger. As a first-aid provider, you may never need to rescue a person. That's because most injured people can stay where they are until emergency personnel arrive. Only when there's an immediate hazard does rescue become necessary, and those instances are uncommon. Even a person who remains in a vehicle after an accident is probably safe; despite what most people think, fire is rare after a car crash and most cars remain upright.

In most cases, moving someone who is injured will likely make the situation worse. In some instances — for example, with a spinal cord injury — moving a person could mean his or her death. Victims with spinal cord injuries should never be moved unless the situation is dire, and then they need to be moved using special techniques to help prevent further injury. (The section, "All the Right Moves," which is later in this chapter, covers this in more detail.)

When is a move a must?

So what are the situations where rescue may be necessary? They include the following:

- ✔ Fire or the possibility of a fire
- ✔ Possibility of explosion
- ✔ Electrical hazards
- ✔ Risk of drowning
- ✔ Extreme temperatures (too hot or too cold)
- ✔ A dangerous accident scene (too much traffic or an unstable building, for example)
- ✔ The need to get to another person who is injured

If the victim isn't facing one of these situations, sit tight and wait for the emergency medical system (EMS) to go into action. Just think of it this way: The emergency crew is going to move the person when they arrive, so it makes little sense to risk further injury by moving him or her only part of the way in the meantime.

If you're forced to make a move

Once again, don't move someone who's been injured unless you have no choice. That said, if you're going to move a person, a few guidelines should be kept in mind:

- ✔ First, activate the emergency medical system. This means calling 911, or your local emergency personnel, and asking for help. If there's time, do it yourself. If not, send someone for help. (You can read more about this in Chapter 6.)

- ✔ *Remember:* Don't move someone who may have a spinal cord injury unless it is absolutely, positively necessary. Signs of an injury include the inability to wiggle fingers or toes, the inability to squeeze your hand, and an upward curl of the toes when the bottom of the foot is stroked. (See Chapter 4 for more on spinal cord injury evaluation.)

- ✔ As long as the person isn't in immediate danger, practice first aid *before* you make the move. This means that you should make sure the person's airways are open, bandage any wounds, and stabilize any broken bones or other injuries as best you can before attempting to get the person to a safe location.

✔ Don't move someone with a head or back injury or someone who has a fractured pelvis, leg, or thigh in an upright position. These injuries must be stabilized and the person should be lying down before transport can occur.

✔ Figure out where you're going. Don't pick up a person before you think about where you're going to put him or her down. Make sure there's a safe location available.

✔ Tell the person where you're going. This goes back to your responsibility to let the victim know at all times what's going on and also helps calm and reassure.

✔ Use teamwork. If other people are around and you're the most competent in terms of first aid, take charge and get them to help you with the rescue. The more hands, the better, so take the opportunity to give some orders — including what they *shouldn't* do with the victim. Don't try to do it all yourself.

✔ When you go into action, move the person as carefully and gently as possible. The body should be kept in a straight line during the move with the head, shoulders, back, and legs all in a row. Also, avoid putting pressure on any one area of the body during a move because the tension can cause further injury.

This may sound simple, but experts agree that lifting and carrying someone is hard to do, especially if you've never done it before. If you're taking a first-aid class, this is a skill you'll want to practice. You may even practice at the scene of an accident — perhaps by moving an uninjured bystander — if there's time to spare.

All the Right Moves

There's a right way and a wrong way to move an injured person, and the technique you use depends on the type of injury, the situation the person is in, and the number of people you have to help you. Here are some of the basic techniques used to get someone from one place to another.

The shoulder drag

This is just what it sounds like. The drag is appropriate for rescuers who are alone and victims who can't walk. It's also one of the safer options for people with spinal cord injuries who *must* be moved. The drag can be done regardless of whether the person is face down or face up. It's especially good when the surrounding area is rough, because it gets the victim's head up off the ground.

Take hold of the person's shirt or coat at the shoulders and brace the head and neck between your forearms to stabilize him and reduce the risk of injury (see Figure 7-1). Then slowly walk backward, pulling the person so that the head, torso, and legs remain in a straight line — don't pull sideways. Also make sure that the garment you're using as a handhold isn't choking the person as you pull. In fact, if there's no risk of spinal cord injury, first place the person on a blanket or coat and then hold on to that as you drag.

When you're picking up a heavy box, the catch phrase is always "Lift with your legs, not with your back," in order to avoid straining your back. Well, that's the catch phrase here, too. When pulling, bend your knees, keep your back straight, and let the muscles in your legs (*not* your back) do most of the work. Bending your knees also means that you won't have to contort yourself into a strange position to do this move.

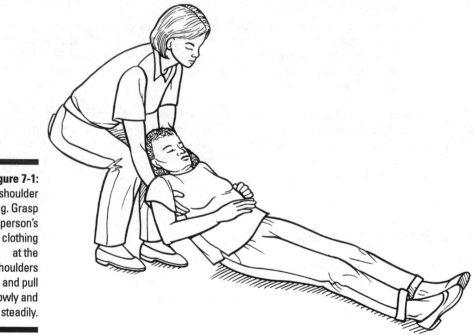

Figure 7-1:
The shoulder drag. Grasp the person's clothing at the shoulders and pull slowly and steadily.

The ankle drag

The shoulder drag is the best choice for people with potential spinal injuries who must be moved or when a rough surface needs to be crossed. However, if the area is smooth and the person has no sign of a dangerous injury, the ankle drag may be used. This means simply taking the person by the ankles and dragging them to safety (see Figure 7-2).

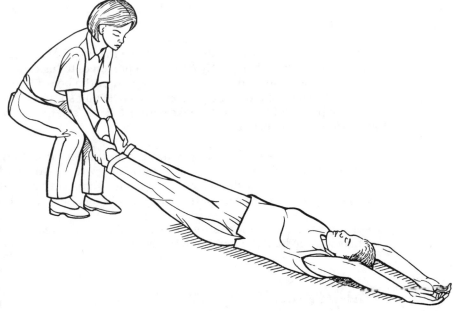

Figure 7-2: The ankle drag. Grasp the person by the ankles and pull slowly and steadily.

Rescue with a board

The shoulder drag is a way to move a spinal cord injury victim when you're alone. If you have help, however, you can use this technique to help minimize further spinal cord injury. You will need a flat, body-length board for this method. First-aid "back boards" are available, but any rigid board will do, whether it's a strong piece of plywood or an old door.

This move seems simple, but it really requires coordination. If possible, leave it up to emergency personnel. And don't attempt it yourself unless you've had proper training.

If the person is lying on one side, simply place the board at an angle parallel to the victim's back. Then gently *log-roll* the person onto his or her back onto the board while supporting the head. Gently lower the board to the ground. (To log-roll means to move the person as a single unit so that the spine is not twisted or bent.) While you roll, make sure the victim's entire body, from head to foot, is supported.

If the person is already lying flat, you need to lift the person onto the board as a unit. Before you do so, use a pillow or blanket wrapped around the neck to stabilize the head and shoulders. You can also support these areas with your hands (one on each side of the head) if nothing else is available.

When lifting the board, make sure that the victim's body stays in position. You may want to bind the person to the board to prevent movement.

One-person support

This move is good if you're alone and you're working with a person without a spinal injury who has one good leg. Essentially, you're providing support while the person limps or walks. Get the victim on his or her feet, and then take your place on the injured side, and put your arm around the waist (see Figure 7-3). Hold the person against your side, and have him or her put an arm over your shoulder for more support.

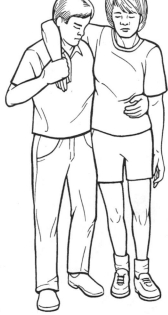

Figure 7-3:
One-person
support.
Support the
victim on
the injured
side by
putting your
arm around
the waist.

One-person carry

When a person (without a spinal injury) who needs to be moved can't walk
and you're alone, you need to perform the one-person carry. Have the person
place an arm around your shoulders. Then pick the person up by placing one
of your arms around the back and another behind the knees and lifting (see
Figure 7-4). This technique is also sometimes called the "cradle carry"
because you're cradling the person in your arms.

Another way to carry a person is the fireman's carry, which is when the
victim is held face down over your shoulder. The fireman's carry is better
than the cradle carry for long distances, but it's rough on the victim and
should only be used when injuries permit.

Another option is the pack-strap carry. In this move, you stand in front of the
victim so that he or she is facing your back. Then draw the arms of the
injured person around your neck and lift the person's body so that it's
against the length of your back. The pack-strap carry is a little easier on the
victim than the fireman's carry is. You can also use the traditional piggy-back
method, which is good for people who can hold on but who can't walk.

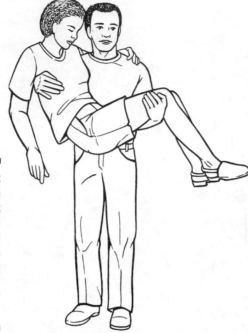

Figure 7-4:
One-person
carry. Pick
the person
up, placing
one arm
behind the
back and
one under
the knees.

Two-person support

This is a variation of the one-person support but uses one person on each side of the victim for support. Again, this technique is good for people who can walk with assistance. See Figure 7-5 for an illustration of this support.

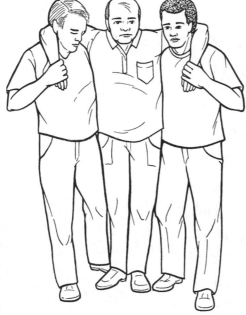

Figure 7-5: If two people are on hand, the victim can be supported between them.

Two-person seat

Two people can carry an injured person in several different ways, but the two-person seat may be the easiest, and it doesn't require any equipment. To perform, grasp one of your own wrists and one wrist of your partner and have your partner do the same. This will form a square seat. Have the victim sit on the seat between the two of you and put his or her arms around your necks (see Figure 7-6). This method, of course, works best for people who are unable to walk but are able to hold on with the arms. It's *not* for people with potential spinal cord injuries.

If a person is unable to hold on, you can use the extremity carry. You or your partner should wrap your arms around the victim's chest under the arms. The other person should stand between the victim's legs, facing the feet, and grip just below the knees. Together, you should be able to lift and carry the person to safety.

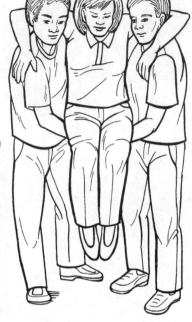

Figure 7-6:
Two-person
seat.
Grasping
each other's
wrists forms
a seat for a
victim who
cannot
walk.

TIP

A chair, if it's handy (and a sturdy one), can also be used in a two-person carry. Simply seat the person on the chair and carry it by its back and legs at a slight angle so that the person doesn't topple out (see Figure 7-7). The chair method is effective and simple and ideal for narrow spaces, such as stairwells and hallways. Keep in mind that people with head and neck injuries or pelvic or leg fractures shouldn't be transported in an upright position.

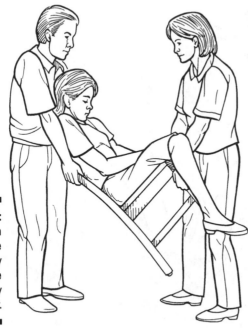

Figure 7-7:
A victim can easily be carried by two people in a sturdy chair.

The blanket lift

If a blanket is available, it can be used as an improvised stretcher to move a victim to safety. The blanket carry shouldn't be used for someone with a potential spinal injury unless you have no other option.

Here's a trick for getting a person onto a blanket with minimal movement, which works especially well if you have someone else help you. Start by folding the blanket into a loose accordion of about four parts. Place the edge of the blanket up against the person's side. Then log-roll the person onto his or her side, being especially careful to support the head and neck and any injured areas. With the person elevated, slide the folded blanket under the body. Then lay the person down again and log-roll in the other direction. Unfold the blanket underneath the person and pull it through. The person should be in the center of the blanket.

The edges of the blanket can then be rolled until the injured person is held snugly within. The rolled edges also make good handholds. Ideally, a person should be supported at the shoulders, lower back, and feet when being lifted. Another person should hold the head steady (see Figure 7-8).

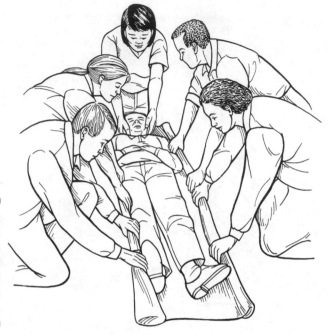

Figure 7-8:
Rescuers
can use the
rolled edges
as hand-
holds in the
blanket lift.

The hammock carry

The hammock carry is a technique for three to six rescuers and a victim (face up or face down) without a spinal cord injury.

When three people are helping, two should kneel on one side of the person (at the head and feet), the third on the other side (in the middle). The rescuer closest to the head should support that area with one arm and put the other arm under the victim's back. The middle rescuer should place one hand between the first rescuer's hands and the other below the buttocks. Finally, the third rescuer should have one hand placed under the buttocks (between the middle rescuer's hands) and the other hand below the knees.

On the count of three or another signal, the victim should be lifted to about waist height as the rescuers kneel. The rescuers should then slide their hands completely under the body and join hands with the person opposite them. Once the hands are interlocked, the rescuers should stand up completely with the victim between them. See Figure 7-9 for an illustration of the hammock carry.

The spacing of the rescuers can be adjusted according to their number.

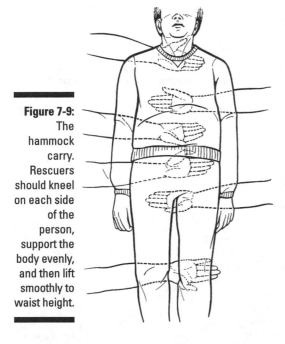

Figure 7-9:
The hammock carry. Rescuers should kneel on each side of the person, support the body evenly, and then lift smoothly to waist height.

Water and Ice Rescues: Getting Back onto Solid Ground

Until now, we've assumed the person you're helping is on dry land. But people are also in danger in and on the water — for example, if they're swimming, boating, or skating on thin ice. Such situations call for a different type of rescuing.

As with any first-aid procedure, call for help immediately before attempting a rescue.

The cardinal rule of ice or water rescue is this: Don't go into the water or out onto the ice yourself *unless there is no alternative.* Unless you're specially trained, don't try to swim out to rescue a person who is drowning; the person could end up pulling you under, too. And with ice, of course, there's the risk you'll fall through as well.

Four different methods can be used for water rescue: the reaching assist, the throwing assist, the rowing assist, and the wading assist. The reaching and throwing assists can also be used for ice rescue.

The reaching assist

The reaching assist involves simply reaching out to a drowning person with a long object such as a stick, pole, or oar. Get the person to grab on, and then pull him or her to safety. Figure 7-10 shows an example of the reaching assist.

If the victim is close enough, use your arms or legs. Even a beach towel could be used to pull someone in.

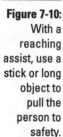

Figure 7-10: With a reaching assist, use a stick or long object to pull the person to safety.

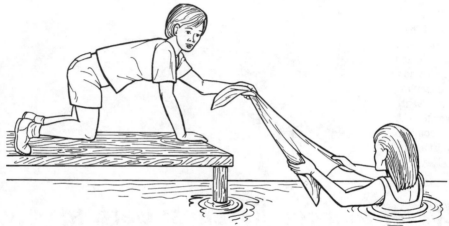

The throwing assist

If the person isn't close enough to be reached with a handy object, throw a floatation device (an inner tube or buoy, for example) out to the victim and have him or her hold on to it to stay above water. If a rope is available, tie it to the object and use it to tow the person back to safety. Figure 7-11 illustrates the throwing assist.

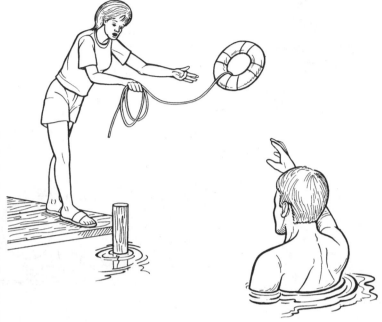

Figure 7-11:
The throw-ing assist. Toss an object that will float to help a person keep his or her head above water.

The rowing assist

If you have a boat and know how to use it, you can row out to where the victim is in trouble. From the boat, throw the person a floatation device or get him or her to hold on to your oar or the back of the boat and row to safety. If you need to get the person into the boat, pull him or her in over the back. This will prevent the boat from flipping over.

The wading assist

In the event that you can't reach the victim from shore and don't have a boat available, you can use the wading assist. This involves wading out to the victim carefully. Keep your footing, and watch out for any strong currents or drop-offs into deep water. From your position in the water, use the throwing assist (see Figure 7-12) or reaching assist (see Figure 7-13) to bring the victim to safety.

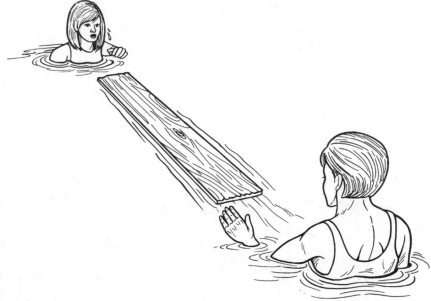

Figure 7-12:
You can use
a piece of
wood or
other
floatable
object to
rescue the
victim.

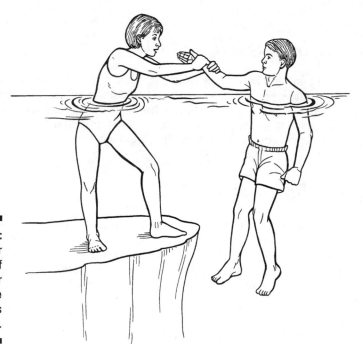

Figure 7-13:
Reach for
the victim if
no other
floatable
object is
available.

If you're using a stick or similar object to reach a victim during the wading assist, remember that you can also use it to test the depth of the water around you.

Ice rescue

In an ice rescue, don't go out onto the ice to pull the person to safety. Instead, stay on shore and use the reaching assist or the throwing assist (using an object with a rope attached).

If enough people are around, you can also form a human chain. In this technique, you should have someone hold on to your ankles. You then lie flat on the ice in order to your distribute weight evenly. If you're not close enough to the victim, another person can form a second link in the chain by lying flat and holding on to your ankles — and having the person on shore hold on as well (see Figure 7-14). For this rescue, inch out onto the ice slowly until you can firmly grasp the hands of the victim.

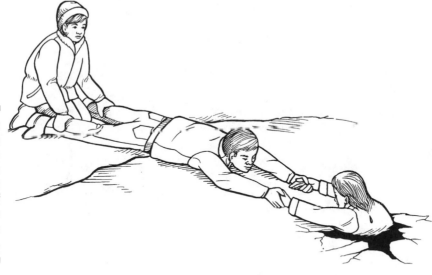

Figure 7-14: In an ice assist, you can form a human chain if others are around to help you.

People who have fallen into frigid water develop hypothermia (an extremely low body temperature) easily. This calls for emergency first aid, which Chapter 16 talks about, and also means the person may not be able to grip an offered object easily. Keep this in mind during an ice rescue.

Part III
First Aid for All Occasions

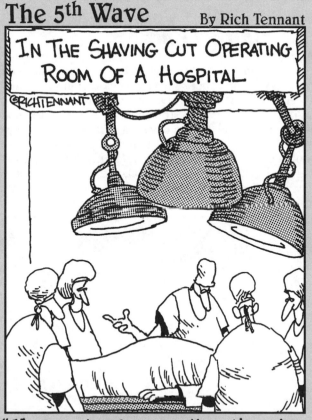

The 5th Wave   By Rich Tennant

IN THE SHAVING CUT OPERATING ROOM OF A HOSPITAL

©RICHTENNANT

"Nurse... hand me another tiny piece of torn toilet paper."

In this part . . .

What do you do if your child has a bloody nose? What if your neighbor's finger gets caught in the lawn mower? This part has the answers, containing information that runs the gamut from stomachache and fever to choking, poisoning, and other nasty stuff. While this book is not a substitute for the opinion of a medical professional — and shouldn't be used as such — the reference lets you know where to start, when to take action, and how to do best by the victim of an accident, injury, or illness.

Chapter 8

Wounds

● ●

In This Chapter

▶ Types of wounds

▶ How to stop the bleeding

▶ Specific tips for specific wounds

▶ Preventing infection

● ●

They say that time heals all wounds, and a little first aid helps speed up that process quite a bit. But first, you've got to know what kind of wound you're looking at. While a *wound,* by definition, is a break in the skin or the mucous membranes of the body, the term also describes internal injuries, even if the skin isn't broken. And there are a host of different kinds of wounds you may come across, each with their own particular first-aid guidelines. This chapter provides a quick introduction to what wounds you might face and how you can take care of them — before you leave the healing process to time.

Types of Wounds

Wounds are characterized in a number of basic ways. For example, when the skin has been broken and tissues and membranes are exposed, the wound is known as an *open wound.* A *closed wound* is one in which the skin is intact, but body tissues have still been injured.

Wounds are also defined by the type of damage that has occurred. Typical wounds fall into one of the following categories:

✔ **Abrasion:** An abrasion is basically a scrape or a scratch. With this type of wound, the outer layers of the skin are injured, but there's little bleeding. An abrasion is usually caused by falling or rubbing against a hard surface — for example, tripping on the sidewalk and skinning your knee.

- **Puncture:** A nail, pencil, or other sharp object may cause a puncture, which is a wound created when a sharp object pierces the skin and creates a hole. Such a wound tends to be small and doesn't bleed a lot, but it may be deep. In some cases, internal organs may be affected by a puncture.

- **Incision:** An incision is a cut with clean edges. This is the type of wound caused by a knife or piece of broken glass. Even if an incision is not very big, bleeding may be heavy.

- **Laceration:** A laceration is a cut with rough, irregular edges. This wound is often caused by contact with a rough or blunt object and tends to be more serious than an incision. Bleeding may be heavy.

- **Avulsion:** An avulsion is a wound in which part of the body has been forcibly torn away. Car crashes, animal and human bites, and gunshots are just a few of the causes of avulsed wounds. These wounds bleed heavily and usually also involve lacerations.

The preceding are all examples of open wounds. Closed wounds occur when tissues or organs are injured, but the skin has not been broken. Signs include a bruise (a collection of blood visible under the skin), bleeding from a body cavity (such as the nose or mouth), clammy skin, pain or tenderness, excessive thirst, and vomited or coughed-up blood. Closed wounds are caused by force and may be minor or very serious.

First to Last

Most wounds are treated the same way: Stopping any bleeding is the first point of order. Closed wounds, puncture wounds, wounds involving embedded objects, and bites require a few different steps than what's listed in this section, but they are described a little later in the chapter under "Tips for Specific Situations."

- Call for help if necessary. Wounds don't always need medical attention. However, if you're dealing with an animal or human bite, a deep or extensive wound, or a wound that won't stop bleeding, call for professional help. You also want to sound the alert if the wound affects a joint (because of the possibility of loss of function) or the face (where there might be risk of scarring), if the victim is in serious pain or is experiencing numbness, or if there is a risk of infection.

- Wash your hands with soap and water.

- Protect yourself against the possibility of acquiring an infection from the victim. That means wearing latex gloves and taking the precautions described in Chapter 3. If latex gloves aren't available, put a layer of bandages or even plastic wrap between you and the wound.

First, stop the bleeding

Here's what to do when a wound involves some bleeding:

✔ Remove any large bits of dirt from the wound. Don't fuss too much with it — the wound will be thoroughly cleaned once bleeding has stopped — but you want to get any visible debris out of there right away if you can.

✔ Apply a dressing (a gauze pad or nonstick pad) and hold it in place while applying pressure. Alternately, you can apply a pressure bandage as described in Chapter 5. Do not put pressure on eye wounds, wounds that have embedded objects, or head wounds that might involve a skull fracture.

✔ Use gravity to your advantage. If the wound is on an arm or leg, elevate the limb above the level of the heart. This makes it a little harder for blood to flow. Remember, though: Don't move a victim who might have a spinal cord injury.

✔ If the dressing becomes soaked through with blood, don't remove it. Just add another dressing on top and press harder on the wound. Resist the temptation to look under the dressing to see if bleeding has stopped. Moving it disturbs the wound and may cause it to start bleeding again.

✔ For minor cuts and scrapes, *Natural Health* magazine recommends applying a topical natural remedy to help stop bleeding. Natural remedies, available in different forms at health food stores, include yarrow, shepherd's purse, witch hazel, plantain, and Calendula. They're said to stop bleeding by constricting blood vessels and helping blood to clot. The herb may be applied in the form of a tincture (the herb soaked in alcohol or vinegar and water for several weeks), a poultice (the herb applied directly to the skin), or a compress (a bandage or cloth soaked in a hot herbal mixture and applied).

If bleeding doesn't stop . . .

If bleeding doesn't stop in a reasonable time — the American Red Cross says 15 minutes — or if the wound is too large to dress with a pressure bandage, apply pressure to the appropriate pressure point. At this stage, you should also seek medical help and watch for symptoms of shock (see Chapter 11). Use the brachial pressure point for arm injuries and the femoral point for leg injuries.

The brachial artery is located on the inside of the upper arm, about halfway between the elbow and the shoulder. To apply pressure to it, grasp the upper arm in the middle, with the thumb on the outside and the flat part of the fingers against the inside. Press your fingers against your thumb, feeling the groove between the biceps and triceps muscles. This squeezes the artery against the bone and slows blood flow.

The femoral artery is located on the front of the body in the middle of the crease where the leg meets the trunk of the body. To apply pressure to it, lay the victim on his or her back (if possible) and place your whole palm over the center of the crease where the artery is located. Keeping your arm straight, lean on your palm, using the weight of your body to provide pressure.

If bleeding doesn't stop, you can place the flat of your fingers on the pressure point, then cover them with your other palm and apply pressure. This method is a little more exact and may give you better results.

Don't use direct pressure if there's a fracture under the site of the wound. This may cause tissue damage and more serious bleeding. Also, don't apply pressure any longer than necessary to stop the bleeding. Lack of blood flow to an area can cause tissue damage. Seek medical help once bleeding persists longer than 15 minutes.

For severe bleeding

If the wound is still bleeding heavily after applying pressure to one of the pressure points — and help still hasn't arrived — a tourniquet might be necessary. Severe bleeding is sometimes called a *hemorrhage*.

Only use a tourniquet when you're facing a life-threatening hemorrhage that won't respond to other treatments. Because a tourniquet cuts off blood flow completely to a limb, the tissue is likely to die and amputation may be necessary. If you're considering using a tourniquet, assume the limb will be lost to save a life. Chapter 5 covers the instructions on applying a tourniquet.

Cleanse the wound once bleeding has stopped

Because of the risk of infection and other complications, you should clean wounds before you bandage them. If you're dealing with a situation where it was difficult to stop the bleeding or you're dealing with a large wound, leave this step up to a medical professional. However, you can clean a shallow wound (no more than skin deep) on your own with first aid.

To clean a wound:

- Wash your hands and put on those latex gloves, if you haven't already done so.
- Use water to rinse out the wound. If you don't have access to running water, use a syringe (one component of a complete first-aid kit) to squirt water on the wound.

- Gently scrub minor scrapes and scratches with soap under running water.

- Rub an antiseptic wipe over the wound. Wipe away from the center of the wound and use a clean part of the wipe for each stroke. Try not to disturb the wound.

- Gently blot the wound dry with a sterile cloth or bandage.

- Apply antibiotic ointment to the wound and bandage it if additional medical help isn't needed. If you can't get the wound completely clean or if help is on the way, cover it loosely with a clean bandage until medical attention is available.

- A number of herbs are considered antibacterial and may be substituted for antibiotic ointment. They include usnea, Echinacea (tincture diluted in water), lemon juice, Calendula lotion (a homeopathic remedy) and oil, or lavender or eucalyptus (diluted in water). These preparations can be bought ready to use at health food and natural health stores. Some people make them themselves with help from books or herbalists.

After the fact

The bandage should be left on a wound until a hard scab forms. If the bandage becomes wet in the meantime, it should be removed and replaced with a new one.

As a wound is healing, examine it once a day for signs of infection. Infection occurs when bacteria or other germs get into a wound and begin to multiply; the result is that a wound won't heal quickly. In addition, some infections — such as tetanus — can be life-threatening. (See the sidebar "Protecting against tetanus" later in the chapter for more information.) Symptoms of infection include

- Swelling and redness

- A hot sensation in the affected area

- Throbbing pain or pain on contact

- Fever

- Pus under the skin or draining from the wound

- Swollen lymph glands in the groin, armpit, or neck

If infection is suspected, consult a doctor. In the meantime, keep the victim still, elevate the affected body part, and apply heat to the area.

Tips for Specific Situations

For most wounds, getting bleeding under control and dressing the wound are the most important points. But if you're dealing with embedded objects, puncture wounds, bites, or closed wounds, you should know a few more pointers.

Closed wounds

As was said earlier, closed wounds are those that don't break the skin. When we think of closed wounds, we often think of small, minor ones, such as bruises and black eyes. These can be treated by applying an ice pack to the injured area. The cold temperature constricts surrounding blood vessels and keeps swelling and discoloration to a minimum. Overall, risk of infection is slim with a closed wound.

But closed wounds can also affect internal organs and body systems and may not be visible. How can you tell if a closed wound is the problem? Look for these signs:

- A rapid, weak pulse
- Clammy skin over all the body
- Pain and tenderness in the affected area, especially if pain seems more severe than the apparent injury would call for
- Thirst
- Restlessness
- Blood in vomit, feces, or urine
- Coughed-up blood
- Swelling
- Discoloration
- A deformed limb (caused by a broken bone inside)

If you suspect a serious closed wound has occurred, call for medical help. Don't move the affected part of the body unless absolutely necessary. If the head has been injured, treat the person as if he or she has a spinal injury. Another caveat: Don't give someone with a suspected internal injury any food or water — even if he or she complains of being thirsty. You'll want to keep the victim's throat and airways clear, and food or water may cause choking.

TIP

Puncture wounds

These wounds are usually deep but are very small in terms of surface area. They're caused by sharp, pointed objects such as pencils, knives, teeth, and the like. Although they don't usually bleed very much, that doesn't mean they're not serious. A puncture can damage internal organs and also becomes infected very easily.

To care for a puncture wound, wash it out with running water and wipe the surface with an antiseptic wipe. Bandage the wound with a piece of gauze or a pad. Do not, however, try to plug the hole with a bandage, and do not put antiseptic ointment into the wound. If you seal off the wound, you're increasing the risk of an infection such as tetanus. (Refer to the sidebar "Protecting against tetanus" for more information.)

Embedded objects

We've all known someone who's stepped on a piece of broken glass or who's gotten a splinter. Those are just two examples of objects that might become embedded in a wound. Other possibilities include a nail, a fishhook, or even the blade of a knife.

If the object is just under the surface of the skin, you can use first aid to remove it. Two tried-and-true methods are use sterilized tweezers to pull out the object or use a sterilized needle to slip in under the object and lift it out. Always pull the object out at the same angle it went in.

If the object penetrates below the level of the skin, leave it where it is — even if it's small. Removing it can cause further damage and trigger bleeding. Instead, have a medical professional remove the object.

If you must leave an embedded object in place, be sure to keep it from being moved or bumped when you transport the victim. The best way to do this is with a ring bandage, which Chapter 5 describes how to make one. Simply wrap the ring to the necessary size, slip it around the embedded object, and bandage it in place. Or you can use a paper cup from your first-aid kit to protect the object. Place the cup upside down over the object, tearing a hole in the bottom of the cup if it's too large to cover it. Then use first-aid tape to hold the cup in place.

All about bites

Bites are open wounds with a twist: an extremely high risk of infection. This is because the mouth of a person or animal is full of bacteria and other germs that can contaminate wounds. With animal bites, the victim is also at the risk of viral infections such as rabies.

In the event of a human bite, clean the wound as best you can and cover it. Then seek medical attention as soon as possible.

Animal bites should also be cleaned thoroughly and dressed, and any bites to the face or neck should be examined by a medical professional. If you suspect the animal might be infected with rabies, make every effort to capture it alive so that it can be examined. If the animal must be killed, try to keep the head intact and retain the body for examination. If the animal can't be captured or properly tested, the victim will need to undergo injections to prevent the onset of rabies. These injections are successful 95 percent of the time.

Making it sterile

Chapter 5 tells how to sterilize bandages and compresses. But how do you sterilize first-aid equipment? For all heat-resistant objects, the best choice is to boil them for about 15 minutes, then store them where they won't become contaminated. If an object would melt in high temperatures, use an alcohol swab to clean off bacteria. In a pinch, you can also use matches to clean small objects, such as needles and tweezers. Just light the match and hold the end of the object in the flame until it turns black. The heat and carbonization take care of any germs.

Warning: Be careful, however, if you're using a needle with carbonization to penetrate the skin. If the carbon gets embedded in the skin, it could cause a permanent "tattoo."

Chapter 9

Injuries

· ·

In This Chapter

▶ Treating the abdomen, spine, chest, and head

▶ Giving first aid for eye, ear, nose, and facial injuries

▶ Handling dental injuries

· ·

*T*hroughout most of this book, you'll find first-aid advice arranged according to the emergency or condition. Sometimes, however, the treatment is directly related to the part of the body that's affected. Here are the basics you need to know when it comes to treating abdominal injuries, facial injuries, and eye injuries, among others.

Abdominal Injuries

Abdominal injuries affect the stomach, the intestines, and the other organs located in the lower part of the torso. These types of injuries are sometimes overlooked because they may be internal and not visible to the eye. For example, an organ may rupture, or there may be internal bleeding. For this reason, seek medical care if you suspect such an injury.

Remember: It's better to be safe than sorry.

Abdominal blow

A blow to the stomach can cause an organ to rupture or internal bleeding to occur. Symptoms include

⌐ Pain in the abdomen

⌐ Bruising

⌐ Vomiting

If you suspect such an injury, first call the emergency medical system (EMS). While waiting for them to arrive, watch the person's heart and breathing rates and be prepared to begin cardiopulmonary resuscitation (CPR) if necessary (and if you are trained).

With any abdominal injury, you should take for granted that a spinal cord injury has also occurred. Therefore, don't move the victim unless absolutely necessary. You should, however, try to prevent shock (discussed in Chapter 11) by covering the person with a blanket.

If the person is vomiting or drooling, a change in position is necessary to keep the vomit out of the airway. In this situation, roll the victim onto his or her side while supporting the head and neck. Specifics on how to do this safely can be found in Chapter 7. Save any vomit for EMS to examine. Do not give food or water.

Abdominal wounds

Follow the instructions provided in Chapter 8 on treating abdominal wounds and bleeding. If an object is lodged in the body, do not remove it — you may cause more damage and make bleeding worse. Instead, stabilize the object and place dressings around it. Do not give food or water.

Protruding organs

A gory thought, for sure, but what do you do if an abdominal injury results in a protruding organ? First, call EMS. Then, cover the organ loosely with a clean cloth or dressing. Pour clean water (water clean enough to drink) over the dressing to make it moist. This will keep the organ from drying out.

Do not use loose cotton wadding, tissue paper, or any other material for a dressing that could disintegrate and stick to the organ when it's wet. Also, do not try to push the organ back into the abdominal cavity. This could injure the organ, further damage abdominal tissue, and introduce germs into the body and cause infection. Finally, do not give food or water.

Back Injuries

The spine is a pretty amazing feature of the human body. It's rigid enough to support the weight of the body and hold it upright, yet it's flexible enough to turn and twist in almost any direction. The reason the spine can do so much is that it's a very complicated structure, made up of a column of small bones called vertebrae linked together with layers of individual muscles. Through the center of the column runs the spinal cord — the rope of nerves that connects the brain to practically every facet of the body.

The complexity of the spine and back increases the risk of injury. It also means you have to be very careful in providing first aid for injuries in order to keep from causing further damage. The key to handling back injuries is this single rule: Do not move a person with a suspected back or spinal cord injury. The only exception to this rule is when the person is in immediate danger — for example, lying inside a burning building. See Chapter 7 for guidelines for moving an injured person safely.

Symptoms

Some indications of spinal or back injury include

- ✔ Pain in the head, neck, or back
- ✔ Numbness and tingling
- ✔ Weakness or loss of feeling in the arms or legs
- ✔ Loss of bladder or bowel control
- ✔ Inability to move
- ✔ Evidence the person was thrown some distance or had fallen
- ✔ Obvious injuries to the face, head, or back

If a person is unconscious and you're not sure if he or she has a spinal injury, just assume that one has occurred.

Signs of spinal cord injuries

Here are some simple tests you can do to test for a spinal cord injury:

- ✔ Ask the victim to move his or her toes or fingers. If they wiggle, that's a sign the spine is fine (which rhymes).

- ✔ Ask the victim to squeeze your hand. Again, any sign of pressure is a positive one.

- ✔ Run a key or hard object from the heel to the toes. If this motion, called the Babinski test, causes the big toe to curl downward, that's good news.

If the toes and fingers don't move, if the person can't squeeze your hand, or if the big toe points upward during the Babinski test, assume a spinal cord injury. That means stay put!

Back to basics

You've heard time and time again about how severe spinal cord injuries can be. But, of course, not all back injuries involve damage to the spinal cord itself — they may just signify a twisted or overused muscle. Painful and annoying? Yes. Life-threatening? No. But it's smart to know how to handle backache when it strikes.

If you're sure that a backache doesn't involve spinal cord injury, try some gentle stretching when it first comes on. Stand up, put your hands on your hips and lean slowly backward, or lie on your back and pull each knee up to your chest one at a time.

Once you've loosened up, apply an ice pack wrapped in a towel every few hours for the first two days after the attack to help reduce swelling. Then switch to a heating pad for a few days to help begin the healing process.

Though it's tempting to take to bed with backache, resist the urge. Rest and relaxation will only serve to weaken your muscles, making matters worse. Instead, get up and around as soon as you're able.

First to last

The first thing to do is call EMS. From there, the instructions turn mainly into what *not* to do. Don't move the person unless he or she is in immediate danger. If CPR or artificial respiration becomes necessary, perform the techniques without changing the person's position. Treat other apparent injuries also without moving the person.

If you must move a person, take care to do it in the right way. Chapter 7 discusses different methods, with the best methods being the shoulder drag and rescue using a board. Both of these techniques offer minimal disruption to — and maximum support of — the injured person.

If the person is vomiting or choking on blood, you may log-roll him or her onto one side. This will help blood and vomit to drain and keep them from blocking the airway. See Chapter 7 for information about the log-roll technique.

While waiting for EMS, keep the person warm and calm.

Head Injuries

When you talk about a head injury, you could mean a problem with any one of a number of features: the scalp, the skull, the brain, and the blood vessels and fluid around the brain. Head injuries can be internal or external. Even if the head isn't cut or bleeding, the brain inside may be bruised or bleeding.

If a person's head has suffered an injury, it's likely that the spinal cord may be affected, too. If there's any chance at all of such an injury, don't move the victim.

Wounds to the scalp

Because of the number of blood vessels in the scalp and head, even a small cut to the head can bleed heavily. To treat these wounds, follow the instructions in Chapter 8, keeping in mind that hair can disguise wounds and make it difficult to tell how serious they are. Also remember that deep wounds may also involve a skull fracture or spinal injury, so don't move the victim or apply a bandage or dressing too tightly.

If a skull fracture is suspected and you need to stop the bleeding, don't apply pressure directly to the wound. Instead, use a ring bandage to apply pressure around the edges of the wound instead of at the center. Another tip to stop bleeding: Raise the victim's head and shoulders slightly to get gravity on your side — but only if there's absolutely no chance of spinal injury.

If there's a chance of skull fracture or brain injury, don't clean out the wound. Contact may cause contamination and lead to infection. Only clean minor surface wounds to the scalp.

Skull fracture

The hard shell that protects the brain is tough, but a severe blow can crack or shatter the bone. Often, skull fractures are hard to diagnose without x-rays because the crack is often small.

Symptoms

Some indications of a skull fracture include

- ✔ Pain in the area of the injury
- ✔ A dent or deformity in the skull
- ✔ Fluid or blood coming from the ears or nose

- Discoloration around the eyes, also called "raccoon eyes" (appears several hours after injury)

- Discoloration behind the ear, also called battle's signs (appears several hours after injury)

- Visible skull or brain tissue

- A penetrating wound (such as a gunshot wound)

First to last

If you suspect a skull fracture, call EMS. Don't move the person, because he or she also may have a spinal injury. Instead, immobilize the head (in whatever position it's currently in) with cushions or folded blankets placed gently around the head and shoulders. Make sure the blankets don't interfere with breathing.

If there is bleeding, don't apply direct pressure to the wound. Instead, use a ring bandage (see Chapter 5) to apply pressure only around the edges of the wound. Don't try to stop any fluid or bleeding coming from the ears or nose, however. This leakage is actually relieving some of the pressure within the skull, and blocking it off will increase that pressure.

Also, don't try to clean a skull fracture because it may contaminate the wound and cause infection.

Brain injuries

The bony skull does a pretty good job of protecting the brain, but sometimes injury does occur. When the head is struck hard, the brain can be jarred and bruised inside the skull. The injured brain then swells, but because it's trapped within the skull, the tissue has no space to expand. The result is increased pressure in the skull and a reduction in blood flow to the brain.

Three common brain injuries include

- **Concussion:** With a concussion, the brain stops functioning temporarily without any permanent damage. No bleeding occurs within the skull.

- **Contusion:** This is essentially a bruise to the brain.

- **Hematoma:** This occurs when blood vessels of the brain are broken, causing blood to collect and harden in a pocket in the skull. The swollen pocket results in an increase in intercranial pressure (pressure within the skull), which may damage soft brain tissues.

Symptoms

You may have a brain injury if you notice these symptoms:

- An obvious injury to the head, such as a dent or bleeding. You may be able to see pieces of shattered skull or brain tissue in the wound.
- Fluid draining from the ears, nose, or mouth.
- Loss of consciousness.
- Seizures.
- Neurological symptoms, such as confusion, disturbance of speech, or change in personality.
- Paralysis in facial muscles.
- Headache that can't be relieved with pain relievers.
- Vomiting.
- Pupils of uneven size.
- Weakness or drowsiness.

First to last

The first thing to do when you suspect a brain injury is to call EMS. Also, take for granted that there is a spinal injury and don't move the victim. Instead, stabilize the head with soft cushions or folded blankets by placing them gently around the head and shoulders, being careful not to disturb the position of the person. Make sure the padding doesn't interfere with breathing.

While waiting for EMS, keep an eye on the victim's breathing and heart rates and give CPR if necessary (and if you're trained). If seizures occur, use cushions or blankets to protect the head and give first aid for seizures (Chapter 19 discusses seizures). Don't try to clean a head wound if there is a skull fracture or brain injury because infection may result.

If fluid or blood is draining from the ears or nose, don't try to stop the flow. This leakage is actually reducing the pressure within the skull — if you block it off, the pressure will increase, causing more damage.

If the victim is vomiting, log-roll him or her onto one side. This helps the vomit drain from the mouth and keeps it from clogging the airways and obstructing breathing. Chapter 7 covers the log-roll technique.

Finally, do what you can for any other injuries the victim might have, such as bleeding. Keep the person calm until help arrives.

Facial and Jaw Injuries

Injuries to the face always require medical attention. For one thing, an injury to the face may also mean a head injury has occurred. But even superficial injuries should be treated because they can cause scarring that may be avoided with proper care.

Symptoms

Common facial injuries include

- ✔ Cuts and scrapes
- ✔ Broken facial bones
- ✔ Injuries to the jaw

If tissues within the mouth and throat are disrupted, the person may have difficulty breathing because the airway may become blocked.

First to last

For serious injuries and broken bones, call EMS right away. While waiting for EMS personnel to arrive, keep an eye on the victim's heart and breathing rates and be prepared to begin CPR if necessary (and if you are trained).

Some facial injuries may make artificial respiration difficult because the mouth and jaw may be injured or deformed. If this is the case, try mouth-to-nose breathing instead by forcing your breath through the victim's nasal passages into the lungs.

Make every effort to keep the person's airway clear. A facial injury can cause blood and debris to get into the throat and interfere with breathing.

Give first aid for wounds and bleeding as necessary. Apply pressure to control bleeding. If you notice broken bones, be gentle as you apply dressings and bandages.

If you suspect a spinal cord injury, don't move the victim — just do what you can with the person in the same position.

If the person's jaw is injured, an ice pack wrapped in a towel may help stop bleeding and reduce swelling until EMS arrives. The jaw may be temporarily supported with a cushion or bandage.

Eye Injuries

Sight is precious, and eye injuries can endanger vision. Be sure to get medical attention for any eye injury, even a minor one.

Common injuries that involve the eye include a blow to the eye, something penetrating the eye, a cut to the eye or eyelid, a foreign body in the eye, or damage to the eye by intense light or chemicals.

Blow to the eye

Usually, a blow to the eye results in a bruise, known as a black eye. In serious cases, the eye itself may be torn or damaged. A blow may also cause bleeding and open the door to infection. While EMS is probably not needed, a person with a blow to the eye should see an eye professional (an optometrist or ophthalmologist) as soon as possible because of the risk to vision.

Penetrating eye injury

Having an object, such as a pencil or a splinter, stuck into the eye is a chilling thought. What do you do if it happens? First, call EMS immediately. Then take steps to protect the injured eye.

Do not remove the object penetrating the eye. Only a medical professional should take on that task. Instead, carefully place a paper cup (one of the recommendations for the first aid kit) or piece of folded cardboard over the object and bandage it into place. This will keep the object from being bumped or forced deeper into the eye.

When you're bandaging the injured eye, also bandage the good eye. This keeps the injured eye from moving with the good eye, which is called *sympathetic movement.*

Cut to eye or eyelid

If only the eyelid is cut, you can stop the bleeding by applying pressure to the wound. Then carefully clean the wound and apply a clean dressing (you can find details on bandages in Chapter 5). Any swelling around the eye can be treated with the application of an ice pack wrapped in a towel. As with any eye injury, seek professional medical care as soon as possible.

If the eye itself is cut, loosely bandage both eyes to keep them from following together. Don't try to wash out the wound, and don't apply pressure to the eye. If there's an object stuck in the eye, don't remove it yourself. Have an eye professional examine any cut as soon as possible.

Sometimes, with a cut to the eye, blood can collect within the eye. If this is the case, you'll be able to see it gathering behind the iris (the colored part) of the eye. Get medical help immediately if you see this symptom.

Foreign body in the eye

A bit of dust, a piece of hair, or some dirt blown by the wind can all cause discomfort if they land in the eye. But irritation is the least of the problems — a foreign object can become embedded in the eye or scratch the eye's surface.

Symptoms

Symptoms of a foreign body include

- ✔ The feeling of having something in the eye
- ✔ Redness of the eye
- ✔ Pain and burning of the eye
- ✔ Headache
- ✔ Tearing of the eye

First to last

If a person gets something in the eye, discourage him or her from rubbing it.

To remove a foreign body from the eye, first wash your hands. Then pull down the lower lid of the eye to see if you can spot the offending object. If you can see it, touch it gently with the corner of a clean tissue or a handkerchief. The object should stick to the tissue and be pulled free (see Figure 9-1). Don't use a cotton swab or loose cotton wadding on the eye.

If you can't see the object beneath the lower lid, ask the person to look down. Gently grasp the lashes of the upper lid, then pull it out and down over the lower lid. This will cause tears that may wash the object away.

If that doesn't work, here's another trick to try. Hold onto the lashes of the upper lid and pull it away from the eye. Then place the stem of a cotton swab or matchstick against the outside of the eyelid and gently pull the eyelid against it. You'll almost be turning the lid inside out for a moment. If you can see the object stuck there, remove it with the edge of a tissue, then flush the eye with an eye cup (another first-aid kit component).

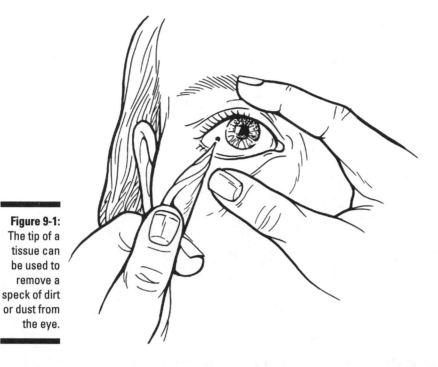

Figure 9-1:
The tip of a
tissue can
be used to
remove a
speck of dirt
or dust from
the eye.

If your attempts to remove the object are unsuccessful, consult an eye professional immediately. And even if the object is removed immediately, a visit to an eye doctor may be a good idea.

Have a sore eye? Then here's a sight for you: the herbal remedy eyebright, known officially as *Euuphrasia officinalis*. Experts recommend boiling a teaspoon of eyebright (along with one of goldenseal, an antibiotic herb) in water. Then, soak a cloth in the cooled liquid and apply to the closed eyelid for relief.

Chemicals in the eye

If a chemical gets into a person's eye, rinse the affected eye and face immediately for at least five minutes. Rinse the eye from the inside corner outward, holding the eye open. This ensures that the chemical won't rinse into the other eye (see Figure 9-2).

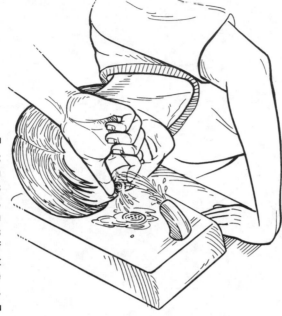

Figure 9-2:
To flush chemicals from an eye, rinse it with generous amounts of water for at least five minutes.

After rinsing, cover the eye with a dry, clean dressing and get medical help as soon as possible. An ophthalmologist — a physician who specializes in the eye — is the best person for the job.

Be sure to get help immediately if drain cleaner, detergent, or another alkaline solution gets into a person's eye. While the injury might not seem so bad initially, swelling and more severe damage may develop through the next hours and threaten sight.

For more information on chemical burns, see Chapter 10.

Light damage to the eye

It seems strange that just looking at light can burn the eye, but just think of all the warnings you hear when an eclipse is about to happen. Eye burns can occur when someone looks for too long at the sun, doesn't use protective eye gear when welding, or looks too long at the glare on snow or at a tanning lamp. The injury might not be apparent immediately. In fact, pain might not set in for as long as six hours.

To treat such injuries, cover both eyes with cold, wet towels and visit an eye professional as soon as possible. Do not allow the victim to rub the eyes, and keep any light from reaching the eyes. Give a pain reliever if necessary.

Ear Injuries

The ear may seem to be a relatively minor part of the body, but it has two important jobs: to collect and help translate sound waves, and to help the body maintain a sense of balance. So without them, you'd not only be deaf, but dizzy.

Common ear injuries include injury to the outer ear, foreign object in the ear, ruptured eardrum, or drainage from within the ear.

Outer ear injury

The outside of the ear is basically cartilage and skin. If a cut occurs, apply direct pressure to stop any bleeding. Then cover the ear with a dressing and fasten it in place with first-aid tape. (Details on applying such bandages can be found in Chapter 5.) An ice pack wrapped in a towel can be applied to the wound to relieve pain and swelling.

If part of the outer ear is torn away or amputated, find the missing piece and seek medical attention right away. There may be a chance the tissue can be reattached.

If you suspect a head injury, call EMS right away.

Foreign object in the ear

Mom's advice has always been "don't put anything in your ear that's smaller than your elbow," and that bit of wisdom holds true. But what if someone doesn't abide by mom's recommendation and something gets caught in there? Here's what to do.

First, calm down the victim and take a look inside the ear. If you can see the object at the entrance to the ear, use tweezers to gently remove it. Have the ear checked by a medical professional to make sure the entire object was removed.

If you cannot see the object clearly, do not try to remove it. Sticking tweezers in the ear might push the object in further, and it might cause damage of its own accord. And don't try to flush the object out with water or oil — it might just absorb the water and swell for an even tighter fit. Instead, get medical help.

If a person ends up with an insect in the ear, don't let the person poke a finger into the ear to try to get it out. You might end up with a very angry bug and a sting to boot.

A better tactic is to have the victim lie down so that the ear is facing up. Hopefully, the angle will help the bug along on its merry way.

If you're sure there's an insect in the ear, a few drops of room-temperature olive or baby oil placed in the ear canal can drown the insect. Then get medical attention as soon as possible to remove it. Don't use oil if the object isn't a bug because oil can cause other things to swell, making them even harder to get out.

Ruptured eardrum

The eardrum is the delicate circle of tissue within the ear that vibrates when sound waves touch it. A blow to the head, an object pushed into the ear, an infection, or a very loud noise can rupture it.

A good sign that an eardrum is ruptured is if you're suddenly unable to hear out of that ear. Pain and bleeding may also be symptoms. In any case, seek medical care immediately. Cover the opening to the ear canal loosely with gauze or cotton to help keep dirt and other contaminants from the ear (which is very susceptible to infection when the eardrum is broken), but don't obstruct the flow of blood or fluid. Also, don't put any instruments or liquids into the ear.

Drainage from the ear

Drainage may indicate a serious head injury (discussed earlier in this chapter). If blood or fluid appears, don't try to stop the flow; the leakage may actually be relieving dangerous pressure within the skull. Instead, cover the ear with a sterile dressing and have the person lie on one side with the affected ear down. Then seek medical attention.

Remember: Don't move the person if he or she has a suspected spinal cord injury.

Nose Injuries

The nose is subject to a few common injuries, namely nosebleeds, a broken nose, or a foreign object caught in the nose.

Nosebleeds

Obviously, a blow to the nose can cause it to bleed. But did you know a nosebleed can also be the result of a variety of medical conditions? These include hemophilia, high blood pressure, allergies, high altitude, and colds. Kids (and adults, too) sometimes get nosebleeds from too much nose picking. Cancer and immune deficiencies also trigger them.

Whatever the cause, nosebleeds are very rarely serious. If one occurs, keep the person calm. Use a clean bandage or cloth to apply gentle pressure to the middle, soft part of the nose, and have the person sit down and lean forward with the head down. Don't ask the person to tip the head backward; this doesn't help stop the flow of blood, and it allows the blood to flow down the back of the throat. An ice pack wrapped in a towel can be applied to the nose to help stop bleeding.

If bleeding doesn't stop or you suspect the nose may be broken, seek medical attention.

Broken nose

A broken nose can be identified by a number of symptoms:

- Pain, swelling, and bruising around the nose.
- Bleeding coming from the nose.
- External damage to the nose.
- Bruising around the eyes.
- A broken nose may look a little crooked, but not always.

First aid for a broken nose means applying an ice pack wrapped in a towel to the injury and having the person sit forward with the head down. The ice will help slow bleeding, while the forward position will keep blood from flowing down the back of the throat. Seek medical help immediately for the person. Don't try to push the broken bone back into place on your own.

A broken nose may mean trauma has occurred that may have also damaged the neck and the spinal cord. Make sure a person doesn't have such injuries before you attempt to move him or her.

Foreign object in the nose

Objects stuck in the nose are largely the domain of young children. Peas, pickles, small toys, marbles, rocks — you name it and it's been found up a nostril. Of course, adults suffer such problems as well, but with far less frequency.

One of the problems with items up the nose is that they can easily be drawn even deeper into the nose by a breath. Another issue is the absorbency factor: Squishy objects can soak up liquid and swell, making them even harder to extract. For both of these reasons, it's best to take care of the situation promptly.

Here's the easiest way to remove something from the nose: Figure out which nostril the object is in, and block the opposite nostril by holding it closed. Have the victim force a strong breath out through the nose. The force of the breath should free the object.

If it doesn't work, try to get the person to sneeze by using some pepper (cartoon-style). If that's unsuccessful, you're going to have to take a trip to the doctor's office, where the object can be removed professionally.

Chest Injuries

Two kinds of chest injuries (both with very descriptive names) usually fall into this category: penetrating chest wounds and sucking chest wounds (which allow air to pass in and out of the chest with each breath). Chapter 20 discusses rib fractures, another kind of chest wound, with bone injuries.

Penetrating chest wounds

Again, a penetrating wound is one in which an object is essentially sticking out of the body. It may be knife, a pencil, or some kind of tool. If this occurs, call EMS immediately.

Do not remove the object from the body because this can trigger bleeding and cause further tissue damage. Instead, protect the object and keep it from moving by placing dressings around it. A paper cup, for example, may be placed over the object and bandaged into place. Alternatively, a ring bandage (see Chapter 5) can be placed around the object and secured.

Keep the victim calm until help arrives and keep an eye on breathing and heart rates. Be prepared to give CPR if necessary (and if you are trained).

Sucking chest wounds

A sucking wound occurs when the injury has penetrated the lung, allowing air to be sucked in and out of the wound as the person breathes. Sucking wounds can be caused by penetrative wounds, gunshots, or other trauma to the chest. Symptoms include

✔ Bubbles in the blood coming from a chest wound

✔ Actual air coming from the wound

A sucking chest wound needs to be sealed immediately to prevent the lung from collapsing. If such a wound occurs, call EMS immediately. Then ask the person to take a deep breath and let it out. Take a piece of plastic, a plastic bag, or a gauze pad covered with petroleum jelly and bandage the wound completely. Seal the bandage to the skin, leaving one corner open. This creates a valve that allows air to escape from the chest but keeps more air from entering.

If the person's condition worsens or he or she seems to have trouble breathing, remove the bandage for a few seconds to allow air to escape. Then reapply the bandage in the same way.

Hand Injuries

The hands are perhaps the greatest tools a person owns. They help people work, play, write, and eat, so they deserve the utmost attention when they're injured.

Because of all the activities that hands are involved in, injuries come from a variety of sources. A finger may be dislocated in a sporting event, the wrist might be twisted in a fall, or the hand may be cut in an accident at work or at home. Here's a rundown of common hand problems and their first-aid solutions.

Finger amputation

Even though Chapter 8 discusses wounds to the hand, it's worth it here to mention more about amputation. Amputation — the loss of a finger — can happen when handling tools, working with a lawnmower, or a number of other situations. What can you do when it happens?

First, call EMS. Then try to control the bleeding using the techniques mentioned in Chapter 8. This involves applying pressure to the wound with a clean, sterile dressing.

And yes, you should also try to find the finger and take it to the hospital with the victim. Take the finger regardless of its condition.

The best way to transport the piece is by rinsing it with clean water and wrapping it in sterile gauze or a clean cloth. The part should then be put into a plastic bag or waterproof container. Then put the container on ice to keep it cool. Don't put the part directly onto the ice because it will become too wet, and don't pack it in ice because frostbite may occur.

If the finger is barely attached to the body — perhaps by a single tendon or flap of skin — don't cut it away. Place it as near to the proper position as you can and bandage it in place. Then place an ice pack on the whole thing.

Bone and joint injuries

Chapter 20 covers these types of injuries to the hand, including dislocation.

Fingernail injuries

If a fingernail is partially torn away, put it back into place and stabilize it with an adhesive bandage as it heals. If the nail is completely torn away, apply antibiotic ointment to the wound and cover it with an adhesive bandage.

If you notice bleeding under the fingernail — usually caused by a blow to the nail — you'll need to relieve the buildup of pressure under the nail or severe pain will result.

To do this, first apply an ice pack to the finger and keep the hand raised above the heart. This will slow swelling.

Then you'll need to do a little "surgery" on the wound. Take a metal paper clip or needle (use the end with the hole) and heat one end in a flame. To avoid burning your fingers, hold the paper clip or needle with some pliers while it becomes red hot.

Once the metal object is heated, press the glowing end against the nail. The clip or needle will go in easily as it melts through the nail; the process is painless because there are no nerves.

Once the hole is made, gently squeeze the nail to drain the built-up blood and relieve pressure. Put an adhesive bandage on the finger as the nail heals.

Blisters

A blister is the collection of blood and fluid under the skin that occurs when the topmost layer of the skin becomes separated from its lower layer. They're caused by friction or rubbing of the skin, often by shoes that don't fit right or use of tools that chafe the hands. (Blisters can also be caused by burns, frostbite, and poison ivy, but those types of blisters and their treatment are discussed elsewhere in this book.)

Blisters should be allowed to heal on their own. You can pierce them with a sterile needle and drain the fluid, then cover them with an adhesive bandage until they heal. Another option is to apply a doughnut-shaped pad over the blister and cover that with a bandage, a technique that takes the pressure off.

Whichever method you use, watch for signs of infection (such as redness, pain, swelling, and discharge) as the blister heals. If it looks like infection is setting in, seek medical attention.

Dental Injuries

A number of injuries can affect the teeth and the mouth and should be treated with first aid. These include knocked-out teeth, broken teeth, and a bitten lip or tongue. Here are some techniques for handling these problems.

Knocked-out tooth

In all but 10 percent of cases, a permanent tooth that has been completely knocked out can be saved and reimplanted — if proper first aid is used. If a baby tooth is knocked out, don't worry about saving it.

Stop the bleeding in the mouth by applying gauze. You can also apply a cool, wet teabag. The tannic acid in the tea helps control bleeding.

If a permanent tooth is knocked out, find the tooth immediately. Handle it only by the crown (the top part that usually shows in the mouth), and don't rinse it or scrub it. Have the victim hold the tooth gently in his or her mouth to keep it moist and get to a dentist as soon as possible.

When you hold a tooth in your mouth, there's always a risk that you'll swallow it. That risk is greater in kids. If you prefer, keep the tooth in a cup of milk or in a special tooth-preserving solution (which can be found at drugstores) instead.

If the permanent tooth or dental work is still partially implanted, don't pull it out. Leave it where it is and get to a dentist right away. Broken or loose dentures should be removed because pieces could be swallowed or inhaled.

Broken tooth

Sometimes a tooth will be broken off instead of knocked out. If this occurs, rinse the injured area gently to remove any dirt or blood. Then cover the broken tooth with a sterile pad soaked in warm water. Get to a dentist right away. An ice pack wrapped in a towel may be used in transit to keep swelling down.

If you can't get to a dentist right away, here's a creative solution. Melt candle wax and mix the liquid with a few strands from a cotton ball. As the wax hardens, apply it to the injured tooth to create a temporary cap. Cover the repair with some sterile gauze.

Bitten tongue or lip

If a person bites his or her tongue or lip, apply pressure to stop the bleeding. You can also apply an ice pack or have the person suck on an ice cube to reduce swelling of the wound.

If bleeding doesn't stop, go to a hospital emergency room.

Genital Injuries

The genital area is full of blood vessels and nerves, and any injury — in men or women — can be very painful. For serious injuries or cases of abuse or assault, call EMS immediately.

When dealing with a genital injury, take extra care in preserving the person's privacy. Shield the area and try to keep the person as calm as possible. Don't let the person walk.

If there is bleeding, use pressure to help control it. If bleeding is coming from the vagina, pack the area with clean cloths or gauze and seek medical attention. And if there is an embedded object, don't remove it. Seek medical care.

Blow to the testicles

For men, the most common genital injury is a blow to the testicles — the very idea of which makes many a brave guy squirm. Though a blow can cause nausea and lingering pain, permanent damage is rare.

The pain felt after this injury is caused by the swelling of the testicle inside its protective sac. The inflexible sac doesn't leave much room for expansion, so the resulting pressure inflames the nerves throughout the abdomen. An ice pack applied to the scrotum can reduce pain and swelling.

If the pain lasts longer than an hour or if the scrotum is bruised, seek medical care immediately. Too much pressure can cause tissue damage that can lead to infertility, blood clots, or even the loss of a testicle.

A word about assault

You don't need to know what happened to a person to provide first aid. However, some genital injuries are caused by physical abuse or rape. If you suspect that some sort of abuse has occurred, call EMS. Don't disturb any possible evidence, if this is the case.

A victim of rape should have a medical examination as soon as possible for several reasons. First, there may be physical injuries that need to be addressed. Also, testing and treatment for certain diseases is necessary. In addition, a medical examination can yield evidence that may help find or convict the perpetrator. A medical exam also opens the door for a referral to counselors that can help the victim deal with the emotional effects of the assault.

Remember: The victim should not change clothes, bathe, or shower before a medical exam if abuse is suspected. Doing so may destroy valuable evidence.

Chapter 10

Beating Burns

· ·

· ·

According to the American Medical Association, burns are one of the leading causes of accidental death in childhood — second only to motor vehicle accidents. By definition, a *burn* is an injury caused by heat, electricity, chemicals, or radiation. Burns usually affect the skin, but they can also cause damage to the inside of the nose, mouth, and throat if a corrosive chemical or hot gas (such as steam) is inhaled into the airways.

Three Degrees of Separation: Telling Burns Apart

Burns are usually divided into three categories: first-degree, second-degree, and third-degree burns. Look at the most serious area of a burn when deciding which category it fits into:

✔ First-degree burns involve superficial damage to the skin. There may be redness and mild pain, but they heal quickly. Common causes of first-degree burns include the sun (as in sunburn) and brief contact with a hot object or liquid.

✔ With second-degree burns, the skin is more seriously damaged, resulting in redness, blisters, swelling, and a wet look to the skin. These burns are deeper than first-degree burns and are considerably more painful. They're caused by severe sunburn and contact with a hot object or liquid, among other things.

Fire facts

Here are a few facts about fire-related injuries from the National Fire Protection Association:

- Every 18 seconds, a fire department responds to a fire in the United States.

- Every 78 seconds, a residential fire breaks out in the United States.

- Every two hours, someone dies in a fire.

- In 1997, more than 3,000 deaths occurred because of residential fires.

- In third-degree burns, a great deal of tissue is lost. The area will have a white or charred appearance, and the skin will be destroyed. These burns, surprisingly enough, are *less* painful than the other types of burns because the nerve endings that sense pain have been burned away. Causes of third-degree burns include electricity, contact with fire, having clothes catch on fire, and sustained contact with a hot object or liquid.

The seriousness of a burn is determined by its rank in these categories and also by how much of the body — and which part — it affects. Adults who have damage to more than 15 percent of the body should be hospitalized. Children and seniors who suffer 10 percent damage should be hospitalized, too.

You should seek medical care in some situations. Burns that affect the face, eyes, hands, feet, genitals, or airways should be cared for by a doctor. The same goes for burns accompanied by other injuries or difficulty breathing. If you're not sure whether to call in professional help, go ahead and call. It's better to be on the safe side.

First to Last

How do you handle burns? It depends on their severity. Here are some guidelines, based on the type of burn you're faced with.

First-degree burns

For superficial burns, immerse the area immediately in cold water or hold it under cool running water for ten minutes. For hard-to-reach areas, apply a clean cloth that has been soaked in cold water and wrung out. If the burned area is large — larger than the person's chest — *don't* try to cool the wound. You run the risk of cooling off the victim too much.

Soothing sunburn

You've done it again. You've spent too much time in the sun without adequate protection, and now you're suffering from sunburn.

Sunburn is caused by exposure to the radiation of the sun. Your skin has a defense against the sun's rays: a pigment called melanin, which absorbs the sun's rays and helps dissipate heat. But continued exposure from the sun will damage cells and blood vessels in the skin. This damage results in the swelling and redness of sunburn. There's also evidence that sun exposure over the long term can trigger skin cancer.

The sting of sunburn can be relieved in a number of different ways. For example, apply a cool compress that's been soaked in milk or witch hazel. Or add a cup of vinegar, colloidal oatmeal (a soothing bath product that contains starch, protein, and a little oil), or baking soda to your bath and take a long soak. Aloe jelly, moisturizer, tea bags, potato slices, and yogurt can also be applied to sunburn for relief. Topical anesthetics that soothe sunburn are also available over the counter. Look for products that contain benzocaine or lidocaine (for example, Solarcaine).

Tip: While these treatments may be soothing, your best defense against sunburn is prevention. On a daily basis, wear a broad-based sunscreen that says on the label that it blocks both UVA and UVB — two different types of ultraviolet rays. Look for a product with a sun protection factor (SPF) of at least 15. And at the same time you're protecting your skin, take care of your eyes by wearing sunglasses that block UV rays. Look for the label "100 percent UV protection" when buying a pair.

Another note on cooling: Don't use ice water on burns, and don't apply ice or an ice pack directly to the skin. Contact with ice can cause frostbite, which damages tissue and may make matters worse. In addition, to keep the wound from becoming contaminated, don't touch it or breathe on it. Also, don't use ointments and salves on the wound — that means no butter or home remedies. (One exception is sunburn, see sidebar "Soothing sunburn.") These will only interfere with healing and contaminate the burn.

Once the burn is cooled, blot it dry with a clean, sterile cloth. Then apply a dry gauze dressing, and skip the antibiotic ointment. Protect the burn from pressure and friction as it heals.

Second-degree burns

With second-degree burns, the procedure is the same as with first-degree burns but with a few important differences.

First, keep an eye out for signs of shock and activate the emergency medical system (EMS) if they appear. Symptoms of shock include a rapid pulse, clammy skin, pale or bluish skin, and weakness. You can help prevent shock by having the victim lay flat, elevating the legs about 12 inches and covering him or her up with a blanket or coat — this position is known as the shock position. *Remember:* Don't move a victim whom you suspect may have a back or neck injury. (For more about shock, see Chapter 11.)

In addition to having the person assume the shock position, elevate the arms if they are burned — this reduces fluid buildup and swelling. If the feet are burned, the victim should not walk.

Finally, make sure the victim gets medical help. You don't need to call EMS unless shock sets in or unless the airway is burned, but a medical professional should treat such burns.

As the burn heals, watch for signs of infection, such as redness, increased pain, and swelling. If blisters form (a symptom of second-degree burn), don't disturb them. Leave them to heal on their own.

Third-degree burns

For third-degree burns, contact EMS right away.

As for first aid: Unlike first- and second-degree burns, don't rinse a third-degree burn with cold water or apply a cool cloth. This could jolt the person's system and send him or her into shock (which was discussed earlier). Also, don't remove any burned clothing that doesn't come off easily. Just leave it where it is and cut around it to remove it if necessary.

Elevate affected body parts, if possible. Keep burned hands above the level of the heart, and elevate burned legs. Victims with facial burns should also have their heads elevated to aid breathing.

Airway burn

An airway burn occurs when a person inhales steam, heated air, smoke, or toxic fumes. Often, an airway burn isn't immediately noticeable and appears in the first 24 hours after the injury.

The problem with airway burns is that they cause swelling, which can restrict breathing. If you suspect an airway burn, call EMS right away. If the victim is conscious, allow him to choose his own position — it's natural to choose the position in which you can breathe best. However, if the person is unconscious, place him or her in the recovery position: on the side, with the top leg bent to support the lower body. Make sure the head is turned to the side and the mouth is open to ease breathing. (More on the recovery position can be found in Chapter 15.)

While waiting for EMS to arrive, cover severe burns with a dry, heavy sterile dressing. As with other types of burns, avoid contamination as much as possible, and don't apply any ointments or salves.

Chemical burns

Some chemicals can cause burns when they come in contact with the skin. If this occurs, rinse the area of contact with large amounts of cold water. If the chemical is acidic, rinse for about five minutes. If the chemical is alkali (drain cleaner or strong detergent), rinse for at least 15 minutes to get the chemical off. If the chemical is unknown, stick with it for at least 20 minutes to be safe. Remove any clothing that has come in contact with the chemical. Once the chemical has been neutralized, treat the burn according to its severity. The categories — or degrees — of burns are discussed in the "Three Degrees of Separation: Telling Burns Apart" section earlier in the chapter.

If the chemical you're dealing with is a powder (for example, dry lime), *don't* add water. Water will just activate the chemical and cause further burning. Instead, brush off the dry chemical carefully, making sure it doesn't get in your eyes or on your skin.

If a chemical gets into a person's eye, rinse the affected eye and face immediately and for at least five minutes. Rinse the eye from the inside corner outward, holding the eye open. This ensures that the chemical won't rinse into the other eye.

After rinsing, cover both eyes with a dry, clean dressing (to keep both eyes immobile and prevent further irritation) and get medical help as soon as possible. An ophthalmologist — a physician who specializes in the eye — is the best person for the job.

Be sure to get help immediately if drain cleaner, detergent, or another alkaline solution gets into a person's eye. While the injury might not seem so bad initially, swelling and more severe damage may develop through the next hours and threaten sight.

Electrical burns

The human body is a great conductor of electricity, and that means any contact with electrical current can cause serious damage.

What happens when electricity passes through the body? Because the body is such a good conductor, the electricity will pass right through all the internal organs and systems. Potential results include loss of consciousness, respiratory failure, or cardiac arrest.

Symptoms of electrocution include

- A tingling sensation
- Third-degree burns where the current entered the body
- Spasms
- Fatigue
- Headache
- Muscle pain
- Unconsciousness

A person also might not be breathing, and his or her heart may have stopped.

Make sure the area is safe before you approach a victim. Then check the pulse and breathing rate. If the person has stopped breathing or the heart has stopped, begin cardiopulmonary resuscitation (CPR) immediately. (See Chapter 19 for instructions.)

Once a person is stabilized, call for help. Place the person in the shock position, on his or her back with legs elevated about 12 inches from the ground. (*Remember:* Don't move a person who might have a spinal cord injury.) Once that's done, treat the electrical burns as you would any third-degree burns and wait for emergency personnel to arrive.

Stop the shock

If someone is being electrocuted, shutting off the current and getting them immediate help are absolutely necessary steps. But handling such a situation is very dangerous because touching the person's body directly or touching the person indirectly via a material that conducts electricity could electrocute you, too. That means you must be exceptionally careful.

Here's what to do: Making sure you're not touching water (water conducts electricity), unplug the appliance the current is coming from, or turn off the house's main power switch — whichever is quicker. If this can't be done, you need to push the victim away from the current. To do this, stand on a dry, thick book or other insulating material (wood and rubber, for example) and push the victim away using a long pole

made of insulating material. (A broom handle would work well.) You could also use a rope or towel to "lasso" the victim and pull him or her out of harm's way. Act quickly, and use whatever materials are close at hand — seconds count! Make sure all your materials are dry to avoid electrocuting yourself.

If the situation involves high voltage current — for example, an outdoor power line — there's not much you can do to help because the electricity is so powerful. Call the power company and let them know about the emergency.

Warning: Don't go near downed power lines, and don't get out of your car if any are nearby. Stay inside until the power is turned off.

Chapter 11

Blocking Shock

- -

- -

The body's systems, in large part, are maintained by the *circulatory system* — the system that carries blood throughout the body to deliver oxygen and nutrients and carry away waste. The circulatory system is made up of the blood, the heart, and a complex network of blood vessels situated throughout the body. The heart pumps the blood through that network to sustain the body.

Shock is the condition that occurs when a part of the circulatory system breaks down, leaving cells without oxygen. Shock is a serious condition: It is one of the leading causes of death for injured people. In fact, injuries that on their own aren't life-threatening can result in death if shock sets in.

The damage that shock causes varies according to the specific injury. If the brain is the part of the body deprived of oxygen, damage will begin in about six minutes. The abdominal organs can go about 45 minutes without oxygen, while the skin and muscles can go as long as three hours.

The circulatory system can be affected by any injury to some degree. Most commonly, shock is found in conjunction with severe bleeding, burns, electrical shock, hypothermia and heatstroke, widespread infection, poisoning, vomiting and diarrhea, and spinal injury.

Because of the wide range of conditions that bring it on, shock is likely in many first-aid situations if precautions aren't taken. For that reason, you should always treat victims — especially infants and children, who can go into shock more quickly and with less warning than adults — for shock.

One note before getting into more specifics about shock: Shock due to a circulatory problem is called *hypovolemic shock,* and that's what's addressed in this chapter. But there are other types of shock. *Anaphylactic shock,* for example, is a severe allergic reaction and has as its symptoms hives, swelling of the face and tongue, and difficulty breathing. You can find out more about this type of shock in Chapter 19. Another kind of shock, *insulin shock,* sets in when blood sugar levels are too low. Symptoms of insulin shock include unconsciousness, hunger, pale skin, sweating, disorientation, and possibly seizures. You can find more on this in Chapter 19.

Symptoms

Early symptoms of shock include

- ✔ Weakness
- ✔ Clammy skin
- ✔ A bluish tinge to the skin
- ✔ A faint but rapid pulse (more than 100 beats per minute)
- ✔ Restlessness and anxiety
- ✔ Thirst
- ✔ Nausea and vomiting

The late stages of shock are marked by

- ✔ Unresponsiveness
- ✔ A mottled color to the skin
- ✔ Dilated pupils (larger than normal)
- ✔ Unconsciousness

Remember: Just because a person doesn't have signs of shock doesn't mean that it won't set in at any minute. In cases of serious injury, treat the person for shock as a preventive measure.

First to Last

The bad news is that once shock sets in, there's nothing you can do to reverse it. But you can help keep its signs and symptoms from progressing.

First, call your emergency medical service (EMS) for help. Then, check to see if the person is wearing a tag with medical information on it. A clue on that tag may point you toward the proper treatment. For example, if a person has a "diabetes" bracelet on, you would know to treat them for diabetic shock. If a person carries a warning about epilepsy, you'd know to provide first aid for that condition. (Chapter 19 covers both epilepsy and diabetes.)

Next, evaluate the person's heart rate and breathing rate and make sure that the airway is open. If the person's heart has stopped or he or she isn't breathing, begin CPR immediately.

Because one symptom of shock is a faint pulse, you may not be able to feel it at the wrist. Try detecting at the carotid artery in the neck or the femoral artery in the groin instead to see if you get better results. You can find instructions on how to do this in Chapter 4.

If the person is stable, place him or her in the shock position (see Figure 11-1). This is simply laying the person flat (don't put pillows under the head) and raising the feet about 12 inches. Use books, a blanket, or anything else handy as a support.

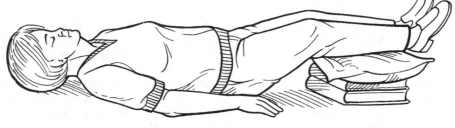

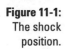
Figure 11-1:
The shock
position.

The shock position shouldn't be used for everyone. Here are a few examples of when it should not be used:

- ✔ If a person has a spinal cord injury, do not move him or her.
- ✔ If a person has a head injury, don't raise the legs for the shock position. Instead, *elevate* the head and shoulders slightly. Make sure they're not lower than the rest of the body.
- ✔ If a person has a face or jaw injury (as opposed to a head injury that would involve the skull) that's bleeding or draining, place him or her on one side to keep the flow of blood and fluid from trickling into the mouth and interfering with breathing. If there's no risk of choking, elevate the head and shoulders slightly as you would with a head injury.
- ✔ If a person has a leg injury, don't move the legs.
- ✔ If a person has a venomous bite, don't raise the bite wound above the level of the heart.

✔ If a person is uncomfortable in the shock position or is having trouble breathing, allow him or her to take the position that's most comfortable.

Once the person is in the shock position (or another appropriate position), begin first aid for any injuries. While doing so, make sure the victim is comfortable. Loosen any restrictive clothing. Cover the person with a blanket to prevent loss of body heat, but do not try to make the person any warmer. Raising the person's temperature may be harmful.

If the person is vomiting or drooling, turn the head to one side to keep the fluid from flowing back into the mouth and into the airways.

If medical help won't be available for an hour or more, it may help to give fluids to the victim. Don't do this, however, if the person is unconscious at any point, vomiting, or having seizures, or if you suspect he or she will need to have surgery or an anesthetic. Also avoid fluids with abdominal injuries.

For adults, give about half a glass of water about every 15 minutes. Children ages 1 to 12 should get about 2 ounces of water every 15 minutes, and infants should get one ounce. Stop giving fluids if the person becomes nauseated or vomits.

The water shouldn't be hot or cold — just room temperature. Adding salt and baking soda to the water (about 1 teaspoon of salt and ½ teaspoon of soda to each quart) will help absorption into the victim's system.

It's very important to keep a constant eye on an injured person's heart and breathing rates. Shock can set in rapidly, so don't assume that just because a person is stable when you arrive on the scene that the situation will remain that way. Continually monitor the victim's vital signs and be prepared to begin CPR if they should fail.

What if There's a Spinal Injury?

It was mentioned above that a person with a spinal injury shouldn't be moved. Does that mean you can't provide first aid? No.

To treat a person with a suspected spinal injury for shock, leave the person in place. Cover him or her with a blanket, and then treat any injuries you can while the person remains in the same position. If the person is vomiting or drooling, however, a change in position is necessary. In this situation, roll the victim onto his or her side while supporting the head and neck. Chapter 7 gives specifics on how to do this safely.

Again, continually monitor vital signs and be prepared to give CPR if necessary.

Chapter 12

Poisoning

· ·

· ·

*T*he U.S. Centers for Disease Control and Prevention have something to say about poisoning. For starters, they report that each year, people make close to 900,000 visits to the emergency room because of poisoning. They also say that most poisonings happen right where you live. That's right: 91 percent of them happen while you're home sweet home. What's more, most poisonings involve children. Kids under the age of 6 account for 53 percent of all cases.

All these numbers add up to a definite need to know what to do should you come face to face with an occurrence of poisoning. And the best way to start that education is with an understanding of what poison is and what it does.

What Is Poison?

A *poison* is any substance that causes damage when introduced into the body. Poisons come in many forms — liquid, gas, and solid — and therefore can get into the body tissues in many different ways. Poisonous gases may be inhaled, while liquids and solids may be swallowed or absorbed through the skin. Poisons may also be injected into the body, perhaps by a syringe or perhaps through the bite of an insect or animal. (Chapter 13 talks about bites and stings.)

Know thy enemy

The most important part of preventing poisonings is keeping potentially dangerous substances out of reach. So what are common household poisons? Here's a rundown:

- Cleaning solutions, including detergent and bleach
- Fuels such as gasoline, kerosene, and oil
- Glue
- Lye
- Poisonous plants, including mountain laurel, rhododendron, foxglove, and nightshade
- Cosmetics and personal care products (even lipstick can be toxic to a young child)
- Pain relievers
- Cough and cold medications

Most poisonings happen in young children, making it imperative that you take steps to protect them with prevention. Store all potentially harmful substances out of children's reach and make sure all containers are labeled correctly to indicate contents. Childproof cabinet locks are available at hardware stores and are easy to install. Also give your kids a healthy dose of common sense by teaching them to stay away from things like detergents and drain cleaner. See the end of this chapter for more tips.

Children, as was said, are the most frequent victims of poisoning. You know how kids are — everything they get their hands on goes directly into the mouth, and that could include a dangerous substance in the area. Among the most frequent causes of poisoning are medicines left within reach of children, lack of supervision of children, dangerous substances transferred into unmarked or incorrectly marked containers, and general carelessness with harmful materials.

Adults, of course, are at risk of poisoning, too — and for many of the same reasons, such as poorly marked containers and carelessness. Other causes of poisoning include drug overdose and combinations of drugs and alcohol in the system. Poisoning may be a method of suicide, as well.

Symptoms and Signs

You've already gotten a sense of how many different forms of poisons there are, and of how many ways they can be taken into the body. So it should come as no surprise that symptoms of poisoning vary greatly, which may make diagnosis difficult.

That having been said, common symptoms of poisoning include

- A rash on the skin or around the mouth
- Headache
- Chills or fever
- Numbness
- Painful swallowing
- Nausea and abdominal problems
- Contracted pupils (this means they're very tight and small)
- Blurred vision
- Shortness of breath or difficulty breathing
- Chest pain and heart palpitations

In serious cases, there may be seizures, muscle twitches, loss of bowel and bladder control, and unconsciousness.

Because of the wide range of symptoms — and the subtle nature of some poisons — you won't always be able to diagnose poisoning using these symptoms. So how do you tell? Here are some signs that might point you to poisoning:

- Information from a bystander
- Signs that a dangerous substance is or was nearby (for example, an empty pill bottle, a toxic plant, or an engine or furnace emitting fumes)
- Stains of liquid or powder on the clothing
- A strange odor on the breath
- Sudden illness or sudden strange behavior
- Depression followed by sudden illness

First to Last

Poisoning is treated according to the type of poison and how it enters the body. First, let's look at what you should do if a person has taken the poison through the mouth. A discussion of how contact with poison should be treated comes after that. Finally, you'll find information on inhalation poisoning and how to handle it.

Don't take our word for it. . .

In this chapter you find some guidelines on typical first-aid treatment for poisoning. However, don't put any of this information into action without the advice of the poison control center.

Every case of poisoning is different, and treatment must be specific to the case. Following the wrong instructions could make things worse.

Poison by swallowing

If you believe a person has swallowed a poisonous substance, first try to identify the poison. Keep the bottle or container that the material came in, or save any of the substance that may have been left behind.

Then call the poison control center for advice. The number for poison control can be found in your phone book with the other emergency numbers, but you can save precious moments by posting it next to your phone now, before a crisis occurs. If you can't find the number or don't have a poison control center in your area, call the emergency medical system (EMS) for advice.

When you call poison control, you will need to tell them:

- The type of poison that was taken
- When the poison was taken
- The victim's age, sex, and weight
- The victim's symptoms
- Whether the victim has eaten anything since taking the poison
- How long it would take you to get to the nearest hospital

The poison control center will give you specific advice on how to treat the poison that was taken. They may give you step-by-step instructions, tell you to go directly to an emergency room, or advise you to call EMS.

Common treatments for poisoning that should be found in your first-aid kit include the following. *Do not use any of these treatments without the advice of the poison control center.*

- **Syrup of ipecac:** This substance induces vomiting, which helps purge the poison from the stomach. If no ipecac is on hand, use a spoon or finger to tickle the back of the victim's throat — it will have the same effect. Ipecac used to be widely used as a poisoning treatment, but now activated charcoal is most often recommended.

✔ **Activated charcoal:** The charcoal binds to the poison and keeps it from being absorbed into the body. Activated charcoal is hard to find in the typical drugstore, so ask your pharmacist about how to get some. Some sources suggest using burnt toast in place of activated charcoal, but this has been found to be an inadequate substitute.

✔ **Epsom salts:** These work as a laxative to purge the system.

While you're providing treatment, remember to monitor the victim's pulse and breathing rate, and make sure the airway is open. If breathing or the heart rate stops, begin cardiopulmonary resuscitation (CPR) immediately.

Seizures, also called convulsions, are marked by involuntary muscle contraction and are also a symptom of poisoning. If one occurs, don't try to restrain the victim and don't put anything in the person's mouth. Do your best to protect the person from bumping into anything or falling. (To find out more about seizures, see Chapter 19.)

Poisoning: What *not* to do

When providing first aid for poisoning, be careful to follow the detailed instructions given to you by the poison control center. Also, keep in mind these general guidelines for poisoning:

✔ Don't give an unconscious victim anything by mouth. It could get into the victim's windpipe and lungs and cause choking or infection.

✔ Don't use a "universal antidote." In the past, it was thought that a single antidote could be used against most poisons. One example of such an antidote is a mixture of ½ oz. activated charcoal, ½ oz. tannic acid, and ½ oz. magnesium oxide in a glass of water. Unfortunately, no single substance can treat all — or even most — forms of poison.

✔ Don't try to dilute the poison with water or milk. Giving fluids may dissolve pills or powdered poisons further, actually speeding up absorption into the body.

✔ Don't try to neutralize the poison unless instructed to do so. Vinegar, olive oil, egg whites, mustard water, and lemon juice are commonly used to neutralize poisons, but don't use them without an expert's advice.

✔ Don't make the victim vomit unless instructed to do so. Syrup of ipecac, which induces vomiting, is often thought of as a treatment for poisoning because it helps get the poison out of the system. But the truth is, acidic or caustic substances, such as drain cleaner or lye, inflict damage on the way down to the stomach. If vomiting is induced, they'll cause just as much damage on the way back up. Syrup of ipecac also takes about 20 minutes to work, and the delay may give the poison more time to be absorbed by the body.

✔ Don't use syrup of ipecac and activated charcoal at the same time. The charcoal will bind to the ipecac and prevent vomiting.

✔ Don't trust the label. Some products offer information on their labels about what to do if they're ingested. Unfortunately, many of these labels have been found to be outdated or incorrect. Call poison control for advice instead.

Remember: Do not use any treatment without the advice of the poison control center.

Vomiting may occur, as well. With vomiting, the important thing is to keep the victim from inhaling any of the vomit. If the person is conscious, have him or her lean over while you support the head. If the person is unconscious, place him or her in the recovery position: lying on one side with the head turned and the top knee and arm bent to support the body. (An illustration of the recovery position is in Chapter 15.)

If the person does vomit, save it and take it with the victim to the hospital. It can be analyzed to help treat the poisoning.

Poison by absorption

A number of poisons do their damage just by coming in contact with the skin. Common examples include poison ivy, poison oak, and poison sumac, which usually strike by causing a local allergic reaction, for example, a rash on the skin. Chemicals, such as pesticides and corrosive substances, also cause damage on contact.

I *really* wish I hadn't eaten that. . .

Something about that meal just didn't taste right, and now your stomach's complaining about it. And you're not the only one: Your companions at the dinner table are also complaining. Welcome to the world of food poisoning.

Food poisoning occurs when harmful bacteria contaminate food that's been left out too long, stored incorrectly, or not cooked the right way. Food in and of itself can also be poisonous: Certain mushrooms and some kinds of fish (when prepared incorrectly) contain toxins.

The most common type of food poisoning is *gastroenteritis*. Its symptoms include diarrhea, abdominal cramps, nausea, vomiting, fever, and headache. Generally, gastroenteritis blows over by itself in about 36 hours.

Kid Stuff: Medical attention should be sought for symptoms of food poisoning — and it should be sought immediately for children and the elderly. The very young and the very old have weaker immune systems than a healthy adult has and require immediate attention if food poisoning strikes. If not treated correctly, death could occur. Precautions should also be taken for those with weakened immune systems (for example, those who are undergoing cancer treatment or who have AIDS).

A more serious type of food poisoning is *botulism*. It's often found in improperly canned foods, honey, and smoked meats and fish. Botulism causes headache and dizziness, which progress to difficulty swallowing and difficulty breathing. If left untreated, botulism can cause paralysis and even death. Symptoms usually set in within 36 hours of ingestion.

Warning: Remember that children and the elderly — and those with weakened immune systems — are more at risk than the average healthy adult. If someone in one of these categories shows symptoms of food poisoning, seek help immediately.

Leaves of three, let it be

Most everyone knows the adage, "Leaves of three, let it be." But whether they know the rhyme or not, many still can't identify poison ivy, sumac, or oak, which cause allergic reactions in about half of all adults. Here's a closer look at these plants, all of which can be found only in North America.

Poison ivy grows as a plant, a vine, or a shrub. It always has three glossy leaves and may have berrylike fruits. The stem may be brown in color.

Poison oak grows as a shrub or vine. It, too, always has three leaves, which resemble oak leaves. Its fruits are hairy.

Poison sumac grows as a shrub or a small tree. The leaves are dark green, and its fruits grow in gray-brown clusters. It can be found in swampy areas.

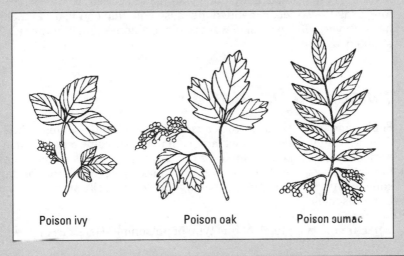

Poison ivy   Poison oak   Poison sumac

WARNING!

After contact with a substance they're allergic to, some individuals are subject to a systemic reaction — a reaction that involves the whole body, not just the skin. The most dangerous symptom of a systemic reaction is *anaphylactic shock,* a severe allergic reaction that causes the airway to swell and makes breathing difficult or impossible. Instructions on how to treat anaphylactic shock are in Chapter 19.

Symptoms of contact poisoning include rash, blisters, swelling, itching, and burning. In severe cases, a high fever may develop. Symptoms usually kick in a few hours after exposure.

To treat contact poisoning, first remove any contaminated clothing. Then rinse the skin with large amounts of water.

If the poison is a chemical or caustic substance, call EMS right away, then continue to wash the affected area with soap and water for at least five minutes.

For poison ivy and the like, emergency medical care is usually not necessary. Just apply calamine or antihistamine lotion to the affected area to soothe the rash and any itching.

Some individuals are subject to anaphylactic shock, a severe allergic reaction that causes the airway to swell and makes breathing difficult or impossible. Instructions on how to treat anaphylactic shock are in Chapter 19.

You can also soothe an itchy rash by applying to it a paste of baking soda and water, or by using the herbal remedies calendula, aloe, or witch hazel as directed on the package or by an herbalist. Adding colloidal oatmeal (a soothing bath product containing starch and protein) to a cool bath before a long soak is also recommended. Because colloidal oatmeal can make the bathtub very slick, you may want to place a nonskid mat in the tub to prevent slipping.

Poison by inhalation

Fumes and toxic gases are the causes of inhalation poisoning. In the most dramatic circumstances, such a poison may overcome a person in a short period of time, making immediate rescue critical. However, many cases of inhalation poisoning happen over the course of several hours or days. In fact, some people who complain of having the flu are really suffering from inhalation poisoning!

What are the symptoms of this type of poisoning? Here's a rundown:

- Headache
- Ringing in the ears
- Chest pain
- Dizziness and blurred vision
- Nausea and vomiting
- Unconsciousness
- Difficulty breathing
- Cardiac arrest

These symptoms may come and go, depending on where the person is at certain times of the day. If pets seem ill (think of a canary in a coal mine) or others in the same area suffer similar symptoms, inhalation poisoning may be the culprit.

The first step to take when dealing with inhalation poisoning is to get the victim to a well-ventilated area with plenty of fresh air. Then call EMS immediately. Make sure they know the situation and that oxygen may be needed for the victim.

While waiting for EMS to arrive, lay the person on the back and loosen all clothing. If the person is unconscious, tip the head back and check to make sure the airway is open. Give artificial respiration or CPR if necessary.

If you discover a victim of inhalation poisoning in a closed space, the first thing you should do is think twice about rushing in to help. You don't want to become a victim yourself, so take a minute to think about what you're about to do. If you notice any discolored vegetation or dead animals in the area, it's a good indication poison is in the area and you're in danger. If you feel you must go, call EMS (or have someone else call) before you venture inside. Don't risk going in if you're alone; make sure there's someone watching out for you in case you get into trouble.

If you do go in, take a deep breath and hold it while you're inside the room. While holding your breath will protect you against inhalation poisoning, it unfortunately won't keep you from being contaminated through the eyes or skin. Use the clothes drag technique (described in Chapter 7) to pull the victim quickly and safely from the area.

Carbon monoxide: A silent killer

It has no smell and no taste, but it causes more deaths each year in the United States than any other toxin. Carbon monoxide is produced when natural gas, coal, wood, kerosene, or other fuels aren't burned completely or adequately ventilated by appliances such as gas dryers and furnaces.

Only a few minutes of exposure to carbon monoxide can trigger symptoms of inhalation poisoning. Breathing an air concentration of a mere 0.05 percent of the gas can be fatal within half an hour.

Tip: To prevent carbon monoxide poisoning, have your furnace inspected annually, and use heaters in well-ventilated areas. Don't use grills in the house, garage, or an enclosed porch. And don't heat up your car in the closed garage, especially if the garage is attached to the house. It's a good idea to invest in at least one carbon monoxide detector, as well: If a problem does occur, the device sounds to alert you to the otherwise undetectable gas. If you suspect carbon monoxide is present, leave the premises and call the police or EMS right away.

Preventing Accidental Poisoning

Take it upon yourself to make your household a little safer by practicing prevention when it comes to poisoning. Here are some tips:

- Keep all harmful products out of reach of children. Store substances on high shelves or in locked cabinets.

- Store materials in their original or well-marked containers.

- Put substances you're using right away after using them. Don't leave the bottle even briefly on a countertop where a child can reach it.

- Buy medicines and other products with childproof caps.

- Read labels before taking or giving medications.

- Safely discard old substances and medications — don't just toss them in the wastebasket.

- Watch for harmful substances you might not suspect. These include liquor, over-the-counter-medications, cosmetics, houseplants, and bug spray.

- Check your home for peeling paint. Older paint may contain lead, which is toxic.

But human concoctions and chemicals aren't the only culprits when it comes to poisoning. The next chapter covers some of the creepy crawlies — spiders, scorpions, snakes, and the like — that call for caution.

Chapter 13

Bites and Stings

. . . .

. . . .

*B*eing outdoors with nature has its perks. You've got sunny skies, green fields, and roaring oceans. Of course, nature has its downside, too, in the form of biting or stinging creatures. After all, you won't find a sky without mosquitoes, a field without ticks, or a sea without jellyfish.

Bites and stings are usually pretty minor, but there's always the risk that infection will occur if they're not properly treated. And then there are rare cases involving poisonous snakes or other critters — another reason to be well-versed in first aid.

Here's a look at different techniques for bites and stings, arranged according to the offending creature. *Note:* You won't find dog or animal bites in this section; they're handled in Chapter 8, with wounds.

Insect Stings

Insects that sting include wasps, hornets, bees, yellow jackets, and fire ants. For most people, being stung results in a local reaction: redness, a little swelling, and some pain at the site of the sting. In others, a sting can mean *anaphylactic shock,* a severe allergic reaction that may make it difficult or impossible to breathe.

Symptoms

Symptoms of allergic reaction include

- ✔ Itching
- ✔ Hives
- ✔ Dizziness
- ✔ Swelling
- ✔ Nausea
- ✔ Difficulty breathing
- ✔ Difficulty swallowing
- ✔ Unconsciousness

First to last

For a local reaction, first remove the stinger if it remains. (The honey bee is the only insect that will leave the stinger behind.) Do this by scraping it away with the edge of a knife, credit card, or another firm object. Don't use tweezers to remove the stinger; this will only cause more venom to be released into the skin.

Once the stinger is out, wash the area with soap and water and apply ice. The ice keeps the swelling down and also keeps the venom from spreading. Watch the victim for at least an hour to make sure a severe reaction doesn't set in.

For pain after a sting, experts recommend acetaminophen or another over-the-counter (OTC) pain reliever. Itching can be relieved with an OTC antihistamine. Natural solutions include a dab of household ammonia on the site or an application of a paste of baking soda and water.

Kids, especially, might need a little relief from the itch of an insect bite. Often, they can't resist scratching the bite until it becomes an open wound. This not only sets the stage for infection but also could cause scarring if it doesn't heal properly. For those reasons, remind little hands to "keep off" those bites.

For a severe reaction, contact emergency medical services (EMS) right away. You should also call EMS if the person was stung in the mouth or throat.

While waiting for EMS, monitor the person's vital signs and begin cardiopulmonary resuscitation (CPR) or artificial respiration if necessary. If the person has allergy medicine, help him or her take it. An Epi-Pen — an already prepared syringe of epinephrine, available by prescription only — is one "antidote" to allergic reactions. Follow the instructions on the pen to administer the medication.

Shock is a risk with allergic reactions. To help prevent it, have the person get into the shock position: lie flat on his or her back with the feet raised about 12 inches. If the person is having difficulty breathing, though, lying down may not be a good idea. Instead, have him or her take the position most comfortable.

Insect Bites

Mosquitoes, lice, bedbugs, gnats, and ticks are among the bugs that bite. These guys don't have venom that might cause an allergic reaction, but there is the risk of infection if the bite isn't cared for.

Symptoms

Symptoms of infection include

- ✔ Redness
- ✔ Swelling
- ✔ Red streaks spreading from the bite
- ✔ Fever
- ✔ Pain
- ✔ Discharge from the bite

If any signs appear, call for medical attention right away. Symptoms may set in several days after the bite first occurs.

First to last

To thwart germs, wash the bite with soap and water. Antiseptic ointment may be applied to aid healing and help reduce itching.

Because of the risk of infection, a tetanus shot may be a good idea for those at risk of insect and other bites.

Ticked off

Ticks are the little creatures that latch onto the skin, bury their heads inside, and drink their fill of blood. But the danger with ticks is not their gory appetites, but their habit of transmitting diseases such as Rocky Mountain spotted fever and Lyme disease while they quench their thirst.

Rocky Mountain spotted fever is transmitted to humans by wood ticks in the western United States. Signs and symptoms include severe headache, chills and fever, aches and pains, restlessness, and a red rash sometime around two to six days after the fever.

Lyme disease is found throughout the United States. In the East, it is transmitted to humans by deer ticks, which are about the size of a poppy seed. In the western states, the western black-legged tick is a carrier of the disease. Signs and symptoms include red rash (often described as target-shaped or bull's eye) at the site of the bite, headache, chills and fever, and joint inflammation and other arthritis-like symptoms.

If you spot a tick on you, don't just pull it off. You may leave the head embedded in the skin, which can cause complications. Instead, get the tick to let go of its own accord by smothering it in petroleum jelly or oil (baby oil or vegetable oil is fine). If the tick doesn't let it go, wait about an hour and gently pull it away with tweezers, being careful to remove the whole creature. If you can't get the whole tick off, call for medical attention. The sooner the tick is removed, the less the risk that a disease has been transmitted.

Once the tick is off, wash the area with soap and water, as you would for any other bite. If signs of infection develop (discussed earlier), seek medical attention.

Spider Bites

Spiders are the stuff of horror movies and haunted houses, but for the most part they're harmless — even if they do bite, their venom is far from powerful enough to overcome a person. However, a few species should be treated with caution.

Types of poisonous spiders and symptoms from their bites

Their names are probably familiar to you: black widow, brown recluse spider, and tarantula. Here are descriptions of these three spiders and what you can expect if you're bitten.

- **Black widow spider:** This black spider is marked with a red, hourglass shaped spot on the abdomen. The bite of the black widow is a quick prick, followed by dull pain within 15 minutes. If the lower part of the body is bitten, you can expect abdominal pain and muscle cramps. If the upper part is bitten, you can expect pain in the shoulders, back, and chest. Headache, chills, sweating, dizziness, nausea, and vomiting are also symptoms.

✔ **Brown recluse spider:** This one has a brown or purplish violin-shaped mark on its back. Its bite causes a painless ulcer that gradually becomes larger, often taking on a bull's-eye appearance. Other symptoms include chills, aches, and nausea.

✔ **Tarantula:** The tarantula is a large, hairy spider. The bite is painful and heals slowly, but doesn't cause systemic reactions.

It is very uncommon for a spider bite to cause death in the United States.

First to last

If a bite occurs, what do you do? First, try to catch the spider — squished or alive — for identification. Then turn your attention to the bite. Wash it with soap and water and apply an ice pack wrapped in a towel to relieve pain and keep the venom from spreading inside the body. Seek medical attention.

Don't try to suck the venom out of a spider bite in imitation of a well-known technique for snake bites. First of all, it doesn't work for spider bites. Spider venom moves too quickly within the system to be removed this way. Second, this method isn't recommended because the mouth's germs may contaminate the wound.

For black widow bites, keep an eye on the victim's vital signs and take steps if breathing or the heart should stop. Again, death by spider is rare, but an antivenin (antidote for venom) may be used for children, the elderly, pregnant women, and those with high blood pressure. Emergency rooms and physicians will have access to this antidote.

Scorpion stings

Scorpions are desert creatures that resemble small lobsters. Equipped with eight legs and a stinger on their long, curved tails, scorpions are poisonous — sometimes even fatally so.

The sting of a scorpion is painful, causing burning around the site, followed by numbness and tingling. In severe cases, paralysis and spasms may occur, and there may be difficulty breathing. Children are at greatest risk for extreme reactions.

Tip: If a scorpion bite occurs, follow the same procedure you would for a spider bite. Watch the vital signs, wash the bite with soap and water, and apply an ice pack. Then seek medical attention.

Jellyfish and Portuguese Man-o-War Stings

The enemy when it comes to jellyfish and its larger relative, the Portuguese man-o-war, is the nematocyst, the stinging device that covers the tentacles of the marine creature. Nematocysts can sting even when the tentacles are detached from the jellyfish — and even when they're almost completely dried out.

When you're in the water, jellyfish and man-o-wars may be hard to spot. Because they have no muscles, these shapeless creatures go with the flow of the water. If you do see one, it will appear as a lumpy, clear, or reddish blob trailed by a mass of slender tentacles, which are dangerous even when detached from the main body. The man-o-war is somewhat larger than the jellyfish, but similar in look.

Symptoms

Stings from jellyfish may cause anything from a slight rash to a severe reaction. Most people, however, don't need medical attention.

Symptoms of a sting include

- Scattered welts
- Burning pain
- Muscle cramping

Pain generally lasts about 30 minutes, while welts can take up to a day to disappear.

First to last

If a jellyfish strikes, first remove any tentacles by scraping them away with a credit card, comb, or the dull blade of a knife. Large tentacles can be removed with a tweezers. Do not rub the tentacles to remove them — this will just make the stinging worse.

Once the tentacles are gone, rinse the area with seawater, rubbing alcohol, or vinegar for 30 minutes or until pain is gone. Diluted household ammonia (¼ strength) may also be used if other materials aren't available. Do not use fresh water to rinse the skin, and do not apply ice.

To further soothe a sting, apply shaving cream or baking soda paste and shave the area. Then repeat the alcohol or vinegar rinse for 15 minutes. Finally, use hydrocortisone cream for several days on the affected area.

Snake Bites

Let's begin this section by saying that almost all of the snakes in North America are not poisonous. (Figure 13-1 shows a map of the risk of snakes in North America.) In fact, you have to worry about only two types of poisonous snakes in the United States: the pit viper and the coral snake. Cottonmouth snakes (also called water moccasins), copperheads, and rattlesnakes are kinds of pit vipers. (Characteristics of these types of snakes can be found in the sidebar "Identifying snakes.")

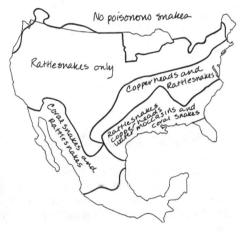

Figure 13-1: Poisonous snakes can be found throughout the United States and Mexico, but not in Canada.

Most snakebites happen when a person is trying to get close to a snake — for example, trying to kill it, move it, or play with it. Less often, a snake attacks in what's called a *legitimate encounter*. A person recognizes the snake and tries to get away from it, only to have it strike.

Symptoms

Symptoms of a snake bite include

- ✔ Pain at the site of the bite
- ✔ Swelling and discoloration
- ✔ Sweating
- ✔ Dizziness
- ✔ Nausea
- ✔ Thirst
- ✔ Headache
- ✔ Difficulty breathing
- ✔ Shock
- ✔ Slurred speech
- ✔ Drooling
- ✔ Delirium
- ✔ Convulsions

Poisonous snake bites: First to last

Traditionally, treatment for snakebites has involved cutting into the bite and sucking out the poison by mouth. However, this method is no longer recommended for several reasons. First, an incision may damage underlying tissues. And second, the bacteria and germs in the mouth may contaminate the wound and cause infection.

That having been said, first get the victim away from the snake. Just because a snake has struck once doesn't mean it won't strike again. (Even snakes that have been decapitated can still bite for several minutes.) If you can kill the snake without danger to yourself, do so and keep the body for identification.

Keep the victim calm and quiet; activity will speed the spread of venom through the body. If you can, carry the person to safety or have him or her walk slowly.

Then call EMS. If you're within a few hours of medical care, get the victim there are soon as possible. As a general rule, antivenin must be given within four hours of the bite to be effective. The time may differ for children or if the snake was very large.

Identifying snakes

With most snakes being nonpoisonous, how can you tell the dangerous few from the rest of the crowd? Here are some pointers.

Pit vipers have a few telling characteristics. First, they have a triangular, flat head that is wider than the neck. Vipers also have oval pupils (like a cat's) and a pit between their nostrils and their eyes. Fangs are also visible, and when the snake bites, one or more puncture marks appear. With nonpoisonous snakes, you won't find puncture marks, but instead a "horseshoe" of marks created by the teeth. To be more specific:

- The rattlesnake can grow to be up to 8 feet long. Its most obvious characteristic is the rattle at the end of the tail.

- Copperheads are smaller — only up to 4 feet long. They have diamond-shaped markings down the body. They can shake their tails when upset, but have no rattles.

- Cottonmouths (also called water moccasins) also get to be 4 feet long. They get their name from the white lining inside its mouth, which shows when the snake is upset.

- Coral snakes have black bands, red bands bordered by yellow or white rings, and a black face. They can grow to be up to 3 feet long. Unlike pit vipers, they have round

pupils, and their fangs may or may not be showing. When they bite, they "chew" their poison into the victim and may not leave puncture marks.

Nonpoisonous snakes have round pupils. They also do not have pits, fangs, or rattles.

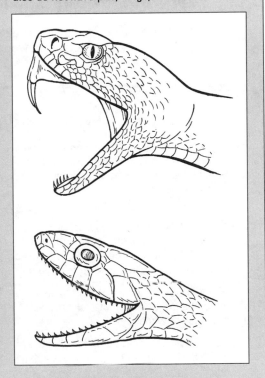

While waiting for medical attention, wash the bite with soap and water. Keep an eye on the person's vital signs and be prepared to give cardiopulmonary resuscitation (CPR) if necessary. You should also be looking for signs of shock. You can move the person into the shock position (flat on the back with legs raised 12 inches) as long as the bitten area itself won't be elevated. See Chapter 11 for more on treating symptoms of shock. For information on CPR, look to Chapter 19.

If a snakebite occurs in the neck or head region, you should still follow the rules and lay the victim on a slope with the head lower than the heart.

However, this probably won't be a concern. Most snakebites occur below the knees (snakes aren't that tall).

If medical care isn't available or if the snake was very large, you can use a special gadget called an extractor. When applied to the bite, the extractor uses suction to prevent the venom from spreading through the body. Look for this device in a drugstore or camping supply outlet.

Nonpoisonous snake bites

A bite from a nonpoisonous snake can be treated just like any other wound. (See Chapter 8 for details on wounds.)

Once bitten, twice shy

For all of the enjoyment nature offers, it can be a bummer when you're bitten. If you're looking to keep the creepy crawlies away from you, try some of these tips:

✔ **Cover yourself:** Long-sleeve shirts, long pants, and high socks and shoes are a must if you want to prevent insect and snake bites. Make sure your clothing is snug at the wrists and ankles to discourage intruders.

✔ **Blend in:** Wearing bright colors makes you more of a target for insects, so stick to natural hues or whites.

✔ **Spray it on:** Insect and tick repellants are worth the investment if you don't want to be bitten — and who does? Just follow manufacturer's instructions when using them to make sure you're not using too much. The chemicals contained in the products can be

harsh and may even damage clothing if used incorrectly.

✔ **Don't be attractive:** Colognes, perfume, and the like not only make you attractive to the opposite sex but also to bugs. Steer clear of these products when heading into the great outdoors unless you want a bee to make a beeline for you.

✔ **Know trouble spots when you see them:** Half the battle in avoiding bites is avoiding the habitats where insects, ticks, and snakes hang out, such as high grass, areas near water, and piles of wood and brush.

✔ **Watch where you're going:** In areas where snakes live, wear high boots and take notice where you're stepping or reaching. If you see a snake, give it a wide berth — don't amble over to investigate.

Chapter 14

Drugs and Drug Abuse

· ·

In This Chapter

▶ Recognizing the dangers of drugs

▶ Knowing what you're up against

▶ Dealing with the consequences

· ·

Drug abuse is the deliberate misuse of a *drug,* a substance that creates a certain response in the body. All drugs — whether they be illegal drugs, legalized drugs (such as nicotine and alcohol), or prescription drugs — have the potential of being misused. Drug abuse destroys lives, takes away self-control, and leads to dangerous behaviors and health complications.

The dark attraction of drugs lies in their capability to alter mood and perceptions. Some people use them to take away pain; others take them to escape from stress and other problems. But drug misuse often leads to *addiction,* a chronic, uncontrollable behavior that occurs after continued exposure to drugs. Some drugs are more addictive than others. Narcotics and cocaine, for example, are highly addictive.

But for all of the dangers of drugs, they can also work wonders. Prescription and over-the-counter drugs help treat diseases and heal wounds, and countless people use them every day. But the key is using them responsibly and according to package directions or a doctor's instructions. Even legitimate drugs can cause overdose. In addition, certain combinations of drugs or a mixture of drugs with certain foods and alcohol can cause symptoms.

Defining Drugs

Drugs, specifically those that affect the mind, can be inhaled, swallowed, absorbed through the skin, or injected. They're classified into general categories:

Inhalant abuse

Drugs can be taken in many different ways: swallowed, injected, and absorbed through the skin, for example. One currently popular way that kids use drugs is to inhale them, a practice sometimes called *huffing* or *bagging*.

Many different products can be used as inhalants, many of them common household goods. Examples include hair spray, whipped cream, glue, markers, paint, and gasoline. The product is inhaled by sniffing it, or by placing it in a container or plastic bag and then inhaling the air within the bag.

Statistics say 7 million children between the ages of 5 and 17 have used inhalants. Yet inhalant abuse is a dangerous practice that kills brain cells and can cause death without warning. Symptoms include nausea, dizziness, lack of coordination, slurred speech, blurred vision, headaches, depression, paranoia, and irregular heartbeat.

If you suspect an inhalant has been used, call for medical help immediately and follow the instructions for inhalation poisoning, found in Chapter 12.

- **Depressants:** These drugs slow down and relax the signals passing through the central nervous system. They're able to produce a physical dependency. Examples include alcohol, barbiturates, sedatives, and tranquilizers.

- **Narcotics:** Narcotics are painkillers that are addictive and produce an intense high. Examples include opium, codeine, heroin, and morphine.

- **Stimulants:** These addicting drugs speed up signals to the central nervous system and produce alert, energetic behavior. Examples include cocaine, amphetamines, caffeine, and nicotine.

- **Hallucinogens:** These "psychedelic" drugs produce hallucinations or changes in the way one perceives the world. Examples include LSD, ecstasy, mescaline, PCP, and marijuana (also called cannabis or hashish).

Discovering the Dangers of Drugs

Initially, a person might use a drug just for an occasional high. But the addictive nature of some drugs makes it hard to give them up. At first, a person might just be psychologically dependent on a drug and rely on it for emotional reasons. But with more use, the dependence becomes physical. Without the drug, the person will suffer withdrawal symptoms such as chills, nausea, fever, and cramps. What's more, greater amounts of the drug may be needed to create the same high — an effect called *tolerance*. Eventually, the person becomes functionally dependent on the drug and needs it for the body to function.

Here are some signs of drug dependence:

- ✔ Changes in personality and behavior
- ✔ Decline in job performance
- ✔ Changes in physical habits, health, or appearance
- ✔ Withdrawal from friends and family
- ✔ Presence of drugs and drug paraphernalia
- ✔ Frequent intoxication

Drug dependence can't be treated with first aid. Treatment usually requires detoxification by medical professionals and a long-term treatment program. But drug abuse can lead to emergency circumstances, specifically overdose (when too much of the drug is taken) and withdrawal (when a physically dependent person is in need of the drug).

Withdrawal

Withdrawal occurs when the body isn't getting the drug it has come to rely on. Symptoms include

- ✔ Aches and pains
- ✔ Chills
- ✔ Cramps
- ✔ Convulsions
- ✔ Dehydration
- ✔ Nausea and vomiting
- ✔ Psychotic behavior
- ✔ Tremors
- ✔ Weakness
- ✔ Loss of consciousness

Withdrawal is a serious medical condition. The first thing you should do is activate the emergency medical system (EMS). If you know what drug the person has been taking, pass that information on.

Once help is on the way, keep an eye on the victim's vital signs. Check the heart rate and breathing rate and make sure the airway is open. If the person stops breathing or the heart stops, begin cardiopulmonary resuscitation (CPR) immediately (if you have proper training).

Otherwise, help the victim to remain calm and comfortable. Loosen any tight clothing and keep the person warm. If the person becomes unconscious, help him or her into the recovery position (on one side, with the top arm and leg bent for support). Don't try to keep the person awake. Also, don't lecture about drug abuse or try to reason with the person. Because of the mind's altered state, it won't do any good.

If the person becomes violent, get out of the way. *Remember:* A person on drugs may not be rational or controllable. Instead of risking your own safety, get help.

In such situations shock is a possibility. Watch out for signs such as blue lips or fingernails, clammy skin, and weakness. (More on shock can be found in Chapter 11.)

If seizures occur, don't try to restrain the person and don't put anything in the person's mouth. Just do what you can to keep the person from banging into anything. (There's more on seizures in Chapter 19.)

Drug overdose

Drug overdose occurs when the level of drugs in the body becomes toxic. It may be a case of taking too much of an illegal drug, but overdose can also occur in innocent circumstances. A person might forget they took their medication and take a second dose. Or they may read the label of the bottle incorrectly. In another scenario, a person might mix a drug with an alcoholic drink and suffer a toxic reaction.

Signs of drug overdose include

- Violent behavior and fear
- Hallucinations
- Sweating
- Drowsiness
- Difficulty breathing
- Nausea and vomiting
- Very large or very small pupils
- Convulsions
- Loss of consciousness

TIP

Too much to drink?

Moderation is recommended, they say, in all things. But having too much to drink is one common excess in the United States. Symptoms are well-known: lowered inhibitions, poor coordination and motor skills, slurred speech, and nausea and vomiting. But an acute overdose may mean more serious symptoms: unconsciousness, difficulty breathing, and signs of shock.

First aid isn't necessary if the person is sleeping and breathing normally, the pulse is normal, and the skin is normal color.

You may encourage the person to sleep in the recovery position (on one side with the top arm and leg bent for support). This position will help keep the airway clear if the person drools or vomits. Vomit in the airway can cause choking. It can also get into the lungs and contaminate them, increasing risk of infection.

You should call for medical attention immediately if you notice signs of shock, such as blue lips and fingernails, clammy skin, and weakness. Keep the person's airway open and give CPR if it becomes necessary (and if you've been trained for it) while waiting for EMS to arrive.

If you find yourself with someone who may have overdosed, first call EMS. Try to find out what drug was taken, how much of it was taken, and when it was taken. Look for clues such as drug paraphernalia, partially filled bottles and empty pill bottles. Then call the poison control center for advice.

Overdose is handled much as withdrawal symptoms are handled. Activate the emergency medical system (EMS), and then keep an eye on the victim's vital signs. Check the heart and breathing rates and make sure the airway is open. If the person stops breathing or the heart stops, begin cardiopulmonary resuscitation (CPR) immediately (if you have proper training). Otherwise, help the victim to remain calm and comfortable. Loosen any tight clothing and keep the person warm. Don't try to keep the person awake. If the person becomes violent, get out of the way.

Chapter 15

Swallowed Objects and Choking

- -

In This Chapter
▶ Causes of choking
▶ Signs and symptoms
▶ First aid
▶ Prevention strategies

- -

Choking is the kind of emergency that first aid is all about. With prompt attention and the knowledge of the appropriate technique, the object causing the problem can be quickly cleared from the airway, leaving the person free to breathe. But if first aid isn't available, death could occur just as quickly. According to the American Heart Association, choking caused by an object in the airway accounts for approximately 3,000 deaths each year.

Choking occurs when a solid object becomes lodged in the airway, obstructing breathing. It often occurs when a person is eating and takes a wrong breath or laughs. As a result, instead of a piece of food making it to the esophagus and from there to the stomach, it gets into the trachea, or windpipe. A good reason, you might say, not to talk with your mouth full.

About two-thirds of choking deaths occur in children under the age of 4. Part of the reason so many choking deaths occur in young children is that their teeth are not yet developed and sometimes don't adequately break down food. Another reason is the tendency for kids to put interesting objects right into the mouth.

People with dentures are also at risk for choking because they don't have complete sensation in the mouth. However, it is dangerous to eat without dentures, so the solution is to eat carefully with them in place.

Another thing that decreases sensation in the mouth is alcohol, so be warned that drinking before and during a meal increases your risk of choking. Intoxication also means a person might eat faster or more recklessly, increasing risk. (And you thought you were safe as long as you didn't drink and drive. Now you're being warned against drinking and eating!)

Symptoms

The most obvious sign of choking is what's appropriately called *the universal sign of choking* — a person clutching his or her throat, unable to speak (see Figure 15-1).

Other indications include

- Desperate attempts to breathe, sometimes accompanied by severe wheezing or crowing sounds
- A bluish color in the face, lips, or hands
- Not breathing
- Unconsciousness

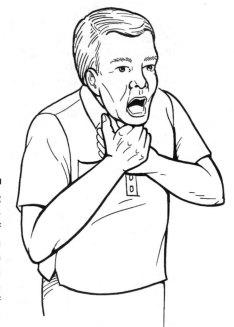

Figure 15-1:
The universal sign of choking can tip you off to someone in desperate need of help.

TIP

Too much to swallow?

So far, the chapter has been about *inhaling* a foreign object. However, it's also possible to *swallow* a foreign object. Swallowing such an object isn't a life-threatening emergency, but it does call for medical attention.

The best thing to do is call a physician and describe the problem. Don't allow the person to eat or drink anything until you've talked to the doctor. Also, don't give the person a laxative to try to speed along digestion unless the doctor recommends that you do so. You may be told to keep an eye on the stool to note when the object has been passed.

First to Last

Adults and infants (under 1 year old) need to be treated differently when they're choking. People who are conscious and unconscious also should be handled differently. Here are some guidelines.

Conscious adults and children over age 1

The first thing to do is ask the person the obvious question, "Are you choking?" If the person can speak, cough, or breathe, do nothing. Allow the person to get into a comfortable position and cough until the object is dislodged. Do not give bread, water, or cough medicine.

If the person can't breathe, cough, or speak, call the emergency medical system (EMS). Then administer the Heimlich maneuver until the object is expelled or the person becomes unconscious (see Figure 15-2). To perform the maneuver:

- ✔ Stand behind the person with your arms under the armpits.

- ✔ Make a fist with one hand and place the thumb in the middle of the person's abdomen — just above the navel. Don't get too close to the lower tip of the breastbone.

- ✔ Grab the fist with your other hand.

- ✔ Push your fist inward and upward into the person's abdomen in quick thrusts. Keep each thrust separate. The idea here is to force air in the lungs out through the windpipe so that the object is expelled.

- ✔ Keep performing thrusts until the airway has been cleared or until the person becomes unconscious.

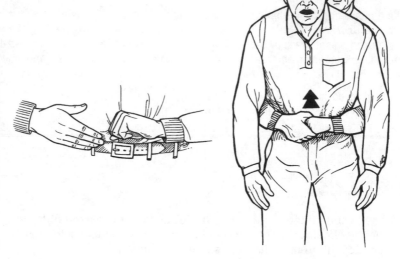

Figure 15-2:
Keep giving the Heimlich maneuver until the object comes out or the person becomes unconscious.

If you're by yourself when you start choking, don't panic — it is possible to perform the Heimlich maneuver on yourself. Make a fist with one hand and place the thumb in the middle of your stomach, just above the navel. Grab the fist with your other hand and push in and upward until the object comes free.

If the person choking is very large or pregnant, use a variation on the Heimlich maneuver. Instead of placing your fist against the abdomen, place it against the center of the breastbone (not on the ribs or the lower tip of the breastbone). Then thrust your fist inward and upward. Continue thrusting until the airway is cleared or the person becomes unconscious (in which case you proceed using the instructions in the next section about treating unconscious victims).

Also, don't stick your fingers blindly into a child's mouth (under age 8 or so). Because the opening is so small, you might just push the object back in again.

Once the person is out of danger, help him or her into the recovery position until help arrives (see Figure 15-3). This means resting the person on his or her side, and then bending the top arm and top leg to support the body.

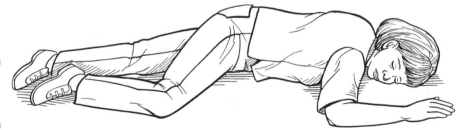

Figure 15-3:
The recovery position.

Even if the obstruction was removed easily, someone who has choked should have a medical exam. Why? Well, for one thing, the obstruction itself or the forcefulness of the first aid may cause physical damage. Another possibility is that the object wasn't truly dislodged, but instead was forced deeper into the lungs. This can cause a relapse of choking at a later time or eventual infection.

Unconscious adults and children over age 1

For an unconscious victim, first call EMS. Then place the person on his or her back. Tilt the head back and see if the person is breathing. Don't poke around in the person's mouth for a trapped object — you could end up just pushing it in farther.

If the person is breathing, stay with the person until help arrives. Do not try to wake the person up, and do not give anything to eat or drink. Keep the person warm, but don't prop the head up with a pillow — the angle may make it harder for the person to breathe.

If the person is not breathing, begin artificial resuscitation. With the person's head tilted back, pinch the nose shut and give two full breaths into the mouth. Each breath should last about one second. You can tell the breath is going into the lungs if the chest rises and falls with each breath. Let the chest fall before you give the next breath.

If the person's chest doesn't rise or fall, tilt the head back farther and try again. If you still don't get results, you'll need to give abdominal thrusts, which are sort of a horizontal version of the Heimlich.

To give abdominal thrusts, straddle the person's thighs. Place the heel of your hand between the navel and the lower tip of the breastbone (see Figure 15-4). Cover it with your other hand and give six to ten quick thrusts straight upward and inward.

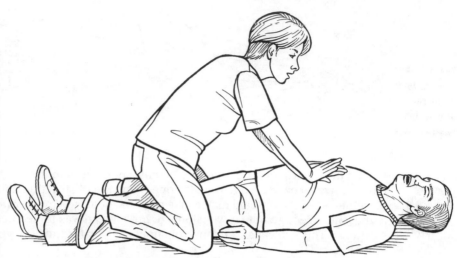

Figure 15-4:
The Heimlich maneuver on an unconscious person is slightly different from a conscious adult.

Then check to see if the object has been dislodged. To do this, do a "sweep" of the mouth: Hold the tongue and jaw with one hand and slide a hooked index finger of the other hand down the inside of the cheek to the base of the tongue. If the object is there, push it out.

If the object is still in the airway, try to give two breaths again with artificial resuscitation. If there's no result, give another six to ten chest thrusts. Continue this cycle until the object is freed or EMS arrives. If the person begins to have seizures, or convulsions, follow the instructions for treating them, which can be found in Chapter 19.

Conscious infant (under 1 year old)

If a infant is coughing forcefully and is taking in air pretty well, don't interfere. Just let the infant get into a comfortable position and cough freely.

If the infant can't cough, breathe, or cry — or if he or she is breathing weakly — call EMS. Don't try to feel for an object in the throat with your fingers. You may just push it in farther.

First aid for a choking infant means giving back blows (see Figure 15-5). Hold the baby face down along your forearm, with the head toward your hand. Hold the head lower than the rest of the infant's body and support it with your hand. Lean your arm against your thigh for support.

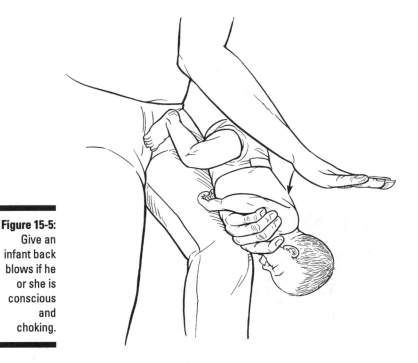

Figure 15-5:
Give an
infant back
blows if he
or she is
conscious
and
choking.

Then give four blows to the back with the heel of your hand. Hit the infant forcefully between the shoulder blades. Hopefully, the blows will dislodge the object causing the choking.

After four blows, immediately flip the baby over with its back against your thigh. Again, hold the head lower than the chest. With the infant in this position, place your index and middle fingers on the infant's breast bone, just below the nipples (see Figure 15-6). Give four chest thrusts, pressing about an inch into the body. Repeat this cycle until the object is dislodged or the infant becomes unconscious. If the infant becomes unconscious, proceed with the instructions for an unconscious infant, listed in the next section.

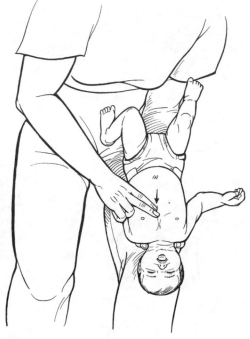

Figure 15-6:
Give the
infant chest
thrusts if the
object isn't
expelled
after four
back blows.

Unconscious infant (under 1 year old)

If the infant is unconscious, call EMS right away. Lay him or her on the back to begin first aid.

The first step is to open the airway. Do this by gently tilting the head back by pushing on the forehead and the chin. Don't push on the soft tissue under the chin, and be sure to keep the infant's mouth open. Both of these measures aid breathing.

Check to see if the baby is breathing. If he or she is not, follow the instructions for infant artificial resuscitation described earlier.

If the baby's chest does not rise and fall with your breaths, give the infant back blows and chest thrusts as you would a conscious infant. Then look into the mouth to see if the object has been dislodged. If you can see it, remove it, but don't stick your fingers blindly into a baby's mouth. Because the opening is so small, you might just push object back in again.

Repeat this cycle until the object has been expelled or until EMS arrives.

A note about drowning

The American Heart Association and the American Red Cross agree: The Heimlich maneuver is not for people who have suffered near drowning, but only for those who have foreign material blocking the airway. This is because the Heimlich essentially creates an artificial cough in a person by pushing on the diaphragm muscle and forcing air through the windpipe.

Tip: So what can be done for a drowning victim? Instead of the Heimlich, rely on basic cardiopulmonary resuscitation to force air into the lungs.

Choking Prevention

Here are a few things you can do to prevent choking from occurring:

- ✔ Keep small objects (such as marbles, beads, and small toys) out of the reach of children. For small kids, buy toys without small parts that may become detached.
- ✔ Keep kids from running or playing with food, candy, or toys in their mouths.
- ✔ Cut your food — and your kids' food — into small pieces.
- ✔ Chew thoroughly before swallowing, especially if you wear dentures.
- ✔ Don't talk (or laugh) with your mouth full.
- ✔ Don't drink large amounts of alcohol before or during a meal.

No matter how much you focus on prevention, there's always the possibility choking will occur anyway. Prepare yourself by taking a first-aid course that includes training in the Heimlich maneuver. Both the Red Cross and American Heart Association often offer them.

Chapter 16

Cold Exposure: Frostbite and Hypothermia

. . . .

. . . .

Say the word *frostbite* or *hypothermia* and people conjure up images of lost explorers in Antarctica, fighting blizzard conditions as they drive their dogsled teams toward the pole. But frostbite can happen in your own backyard, maybe while you're shoveling snow, or even *in* your house, if you leave an uncovered ice pack on the skin for too long.

Understanding Frostbite

In frostbite, the skin tissue has become frozen. In some cases, ice crystals form in the tissue, enlarging as they draw water from surrounding cells. In other cases, frozen tissue may cause clots that prevent blood from reaching other areas. This causes tissue damage. Severe cases of frostbite can cause gangrene (tissue death) and possibly lead to amputation.

The main cause of frostbite is cold temperatures, usually caused by frigid weather and high winds. But other factors complicate the effects of cold. Wet clothing and tight clothing or shoes (which cut off the circulation of warming blood) encourage frostbite. Medical conditions such as poor circulation, fatigue, and certain diseases (such as diabetes) may play a role. Smoking, drinking alcohol, and sitting in a cramped position can contribute, too.

Frostbite most often affects the extremities — the feet and the hands — and the face and the nose. This is because these parts aren't near any large muscles (which produce heat), have poorer circulation than the rest of the body, and are often left exposed to the cold.

Symptoms

Frostnip, a very minor form of frostbite, has the following symptoms:

- Flexible (not frozen) skin
- Cold, pale skin
- No pain
- After warming, a red and tingling area

Superficial frostbite is marked by these symptoms:

- Stiff upper layer of skin, which is soft underneath
- Pale skin
- Pain, aching, or tingling in affected part

Severe frostbite has these symptoms:

- Hard, solid skin
- Pale skin
- Numbness in a previously painful affected area
- After warming, blisters

First to last

The first thing to do is to get the person in, out of the cold. Have the person remove any tight clothing that's restricting circulation. Then seek medical attention. If the person has severe frostbite (marked by hard, solid skin), call the emergency medical system (EMS).

If you're more than two hours away from medical help, you should treat the frostbite yourself by soaking the affected part in warm water. Don't use direct heat, such as a heater or a campfire, to treat frostbite because burns can easily occur. Also, don't attempt to thaw frostbite unless you're sure you can keep it from refreezing.

Use water that's 102 degrees to 106 degrees F, and keep it at that temperature until the tissues are softened. Warming usually takes 20 to 40 minutes. If the body part can't be immersed in water (such as the nose), apply a compress soaked in warm water. A pain reliever can be given to ease pain during thawing. Blood moving back into injured tissues causes the pain.

Use a thermometer (a component in most first-aid kits) to measure the temperature of the water. If the water is any hotter than 106 degrees F, you run the risk of burning the person; any cooler than 102 degrees F, and the frostbite won't thaw quickly. If you have no thermometer, test the water on your arm or elbow.

Remember those ice crystals that were mentioned? They're the reason you shouldn't rub a person's skin to warm it up. Rubbing can push the crystals into nearby cells and cause damage. It's also not helpful to rub the skin with ice, snow, or alcohol.

Once the victim is warm, dry the skin and apply a sterile dressing. If the toes or fingers are frostbitten, put dressings between them. If blisters appear, do not rupture them; just cover them carefully.

Move the person as little as possible once he or she is warmed up, and don't massage the frostbitten area (which might be damaged). The person also shouldn't be allowed to walk. Instructions on how to carry an injured person can be found in Chapter 7.

Handling Hypothermia

Your normal internal body temperature is somewhere around 98.6 degrees F, and your body has a host of different ways (such as shivering when you're cold and sweating when you're hot) to maintain that norm. Hypothermia, however, occurs when the internal temperature drops enough to affect the body's systems. Most people die when body temperature falls to 80 degrees F.

Hypothermia is caused by exposure to frigid temperatures, wet clothes, immersion in cold water, and prolonged periods in a cold room. People with poor circulation and those who smoke and drink alcohol are at increased risk of hypothermia, as are infants and the elderly (whose body-temperature-maintenance systems aren't up to par). People with diseases such as diabetes (which affects circulation) are also at risk.

Symptoms

Hypothermia can be mild or severe. Symptoms of mild hypothermia include

- Shivering
- Urge to urinate
- Stiffness and staggering
- Slurred speech
- Confusion

While frostbite most often affects the hands and feet, people with hypothermia may complain of having a cold back or stomach.

Severe hypothermia involves

- No shivering
- Slurred speech
- Irrational behavior
- Drowsiness
- Skin that's cold to the touch
- Stiff muscles
- Slow breathing and heart rates
- Blue or pale skin

If hypothermia progresses, unconsciousness and cardiac arrest can occur. More than half of all people with severe hypothermia die.

People with hypothermia sometimes appear to be dead when they're not — they're cold to the touch and stiff (as with rigor mortis) and don't appear to be breathing, but they're still alive. For this reason, never assume a person found lying in the cold is dead. Call EMS.

First to last

If the condition is mild, use first-aid measures, then seek medical attention. If hypothermia is anything other than minor, call EMS right away.

Your first move should be to get the person out of the cold. In mild cases, move the victim as little as possible and keep him or her from getting any colder. Have the person take off any constrictive clothing. Use a blanket (another ingredient in a first-aid kit) to hold in body heat, and use your own body heat to warm the person up. You can also apply compresses soaked in warm water. A warm drink is recommended if the person can easily swallow — but stay away from alcoholic and caffeinated beverages because they hinder circulation.

If the person is more than mildly hypothermic and you've called EMS, monitor the person's heart and breathing rates while you wait for EMS to arrive. If the heart stops (cardiac arrest is possible in those with hypothermia), begin cardiopulmonary resuscitation (CPR), if you're trained to do so. If the breathing rate drops below six breaths per minute, begin artificial respiration. If the rate is above six breaths per minute, don't interfere.

Don't do chest compressions with artificial respiration unless you are sure the heart has stopped. Compressions can actually trigger cardiac arrest in those with hypothermia.

A person with hypothermia is also likely to have frostbite. Treat the hypothermia, first, however, when providing first aid.

Had enough of the cold? The next chapter offers some information about heat exposure.

Chapter 17

The Temperature's Rising: Heat Cramps, Heat Exhaustion, and Heat Stroke

Maybe it's a game of badminton on a hot summer weekend. Maybe it's not having enough to drink before a tough workout. Maybe it's trying to mow the lawn when a heat advisory is in effect. All of these are potential causes of heat cramps, heat exhaustion, and heat stroke: three degrees of heat-related illness that at the least could cause pain and at the worst could cause organ damage and even death.

Heat Cramps: Don't Let It Strain You

One of the first signs that you're becoming overheated is heat cramps. These strike when the body loses too much salt due to prolonged perspiration. They usually occur after a person has been exercising for a long period in the heat or hasn't had enough to drink.

Not getting enough fluids causes a condition called *dehydration,* in which the body runs low on water. Dehydration is actually very easy to get. In fact, by the time a person is thirsty, he or she is already suffering from dehydration.

Symptoms

Signs of heat cramps include

- Cramps in the legs or stomach
- Perspiration
- Lightheadedness
- Weakness

A person with heat cramps will have a normal body temperature.

First to last

Heat cramps are pretty minor, but if left untreated, they can lead to more serious heat-related illnesses. The first step in providing first aid is to get the person to a cool place. Have him or her sit in the shade or move into an air-conditioned room. You might also hose the person down with some cool water.

To ease cramps, have the person stretch the muscle that hurts. Don't massage the muscle, however. Rubbing won't help and may make the muscle hurt more.

Once the person is out of the heat, give him or her a cool drink. Water with a touch of salt (about ½ teaspoon per quart) helps replenish the body's stores — the salt helps the body absorb the water faster. Don't give a person with heat cramps salt tablets to ease the cramps. These can cause nausea and vomiting. Drinks with electrolytes, such as Gatorade and other sports drinks, may be helpful.

Stay away from alcohol and caffeinated beverages; these are *diuretics,* substances that encourage urination, so they'll only add to dehydration. They also interfere with the body's method of regulating temperature.

If a child is suffering heat cramps, seek medical attention. While heat cramps are relatively minor, the very young and the very old are usually affected more severely than the average healthy adult. Don't underestimate the seriousness of the problem.

Heat Exhaustion: It's More Than Just Feeling Tired

Heat exhaustion is more serious than heat cramps but not as serious as heat stroke. It occurs when the body becomes dehydrated, or hasn't gotten enough fluids.

Symptoms

Signs of heat exhaustion include

- ✔ Profuse sweating
- ✔ Headache
- ✔ Dizziness
- ✔ Weakness
- ✔ Nausea and vomiting

A person with heat exhaustion will have a normal body temperature and think clearly.

First to last

The first thing to do in the case of heat exhaustion is get the person out of the heat. Use an air-conditioned room, a shady spot, or a dousing with cold water to help get his or her temperature down.

Once the person is cooling down, have him or her sit with his or her legs straight and raised about 12 inches. Remove any excess clothing, and give some cool water mixed with salt (½ teaspoon per quart). Don't give salt tablets, which have nausea and vomiting as potential side effects.

An alternative to salt water is an electrolyte beverage, such as Gatorade. Don't give alcohol or caffeine.

With heat exhaustion, it's a good idea to sponge the person down with cool water. Or you can wrap the person in a wet sheet and turn a fan in that direction. The fan evaporates the water, which cools the person very effectively.

If the condition doesn't subside in about half an hour, seek medical attention because heat stroke may set in.

Heat Stroke: It's No Joke

Heat stroke is a serious condition that can cause death if not treated promptly. It occurs when a person's internal body temperature — which is normally kept in check by perspiration — rises above 98.6 degrees F. Not enough fluids (which are needed to create perspiration), extremely high temperatures, and exercise and exertion on a hot day are the main causes of heat stroke.

Symptoms

Symptoms of heat stroke include

- Elevated body temperature (more than 102 degrees F)
- Dry, hot skin
- Dark yellow urine
- Rapid but weak pulse
- Rapid breathing
- Confusion
- Weakness
- Seizures
- Unconsciousness

First to last

If you suspect heat stroke, or if heat cramps or heat exhaustion become worse, call the emergency medical system (EMS).

Then cool the victim as quickly as you can. This means getting the person into the shade or an air-conditioned room and removing any unnecessary clothing.

You can cool a person in a few different ways. For example, douse the person with cool water, wrap him or her in a cool, wet sheet, and aim a fan in that direction. You can also apply an ice pack wrapped in a towel to the neck, groin, or armpits to help with the cool-down. In very severe cases, you might want to immerse the person in cool or cold water in a tub, lake, or swimming pool. However, only do this if you can keep a close eye on the person's condition.

Don't worry about jarring an overheated person with ice-cold water or a cold compress — there's no harm in that. The idea is to cool the victim down as fast as you can.

As the victim is being cooled, have him or her get into the shock position: lying flat on the back with the legs raised about 12 inches. Watch for signs that shock is setting in. (You can read about shock in Chapter 11.)

If the person loses consciousness, stay with him or her and monitor vital signs. Be prepared to provide cardiopulmonary resuscitation (CPR) if necessary (and if you are trained).

If the person begins to have a seizure, don't restrain him or her, but just provide protection against banging into something in the area. More on seizures can be found in Chapter 19.

Heat stroke doesn't affect only healthy people who've overdone it in the sun. It also affects children and the elderly and people with circulatory problems. So take signs of heat cramps, exhaustion, and stroke very seriously when they appear in people in these categories.

Chapter 18

Catch Your Breath: Respiratory Emergencies

*B*reathing is possibly the bodily function most essential to life. As you know, the body is made up of cells that need oxygen to function. Inhaling brings in that oxygen, which is then absorbed into the bloodstream and delivered to the cells. At the same time, exhaling rids the body of wastes, such as carbon dioxide. If breathing stops — which is called respiratory failure — even if only for a short time, the cells of the brain may become damaged. In fact, experts say death occurs a short six minutes after a person stops breathing.

But an inability to breathe is only one kind of respiratory emergency. A person may have difficulty breathing but still be able to get air into the lungs. Another person may experience hyperventilation: breathing too rapidly. This chapter talks about all these problems.

Causes of Breathing Problems

The brain, the throat, the muscles in the head and neck, the lungs, the ribs, and the diaphragm muscle in the abdomen all play a role in the process of breathing, so it's no wonder that breathing-related problems have a host of causes. For example, an infection might interfere with lung function. If the heart fails, fluid may collect in the lungs. Even a muscle pull might interfere with taking a deep breath.

Some common causes of breathing problems are addressed elsewhere in this book. Here's a guide to where you'll find information about treating them:

- ✔ **Choking:** If an object or liquid blocks the airway, it becomes impossible to breathe. If this occurs, it may be necessary to perform the Heimlich maneuver, which Chapter 15 covers.

- ✔ **Severe allergic reaction:** Some people are prone to anaphylactic shock, a rare but serious form of allergic reaction. When anaphylactic shock sets in, the airway swells and breathing becomes difficult. Chapter 19 talks about treating this condition.

- ✔ **Cardiac arrest:** Cardiac arrest is another way of saying that a person's heart has stopped, and breathing often stops in the same circumstances. As you'll learn, artificial respiration goes hand in hand with cardiopulmonary resuscitation (CPR).

- ✔ **Poisoning:** Difficulty breathing can be a sign of poisoning, especially if it's accompanied by symptoms such as nausea, headache, chills or fever, contracted pupils, and blurred vision. More on poisoning can be found in Chapter 12.

- ✔ **Drug overdose:** An overdose is marked not only by difficulty breathing but also sweating, hallucinations, drowsiness, violent behavior, and nausea and vomiting. See Chapter 14 for more about drug use and abuse.

- ✔ **Chest injury:** A wound to the chest can affect the ribs and the lungs and, therefore, breathing. In some cases, a wound may penetrate the lung itself. This type of wound is called a sucking wound, and it needs special attention — as described in Chapter 9.

Difficulty Breathing

What do you do if someone starts huffing and puffing in your presence, trying to draw a breath? If you know the person has a specific medical condition, such as asthma, treat the condition accordingly. If you don't know the cause, however, don't panic. You don't necessarily need to know what's causing the breathing problem in order to provide first aid.

The nature of breathing problems is such that the person may be unable to tell you what's causing the problem. But one good clue — if there's no obvious cause — may be a Medic Alert bracelet or other token that points to a medical emergency. Asthma, diabetes, heart disease, and more conditions may lead to difficulty breathing, and they all have their own first-aid measures.

Symptoms

Here are some clues that a person is having trouble breathing:

- ✔ Shortness of breath
- ✔ Difficulty taking a deep breath
- ✔ Coughing and wheezing
- ✔ Blue lips and fingernails

First to last

If a person is having trouble breathing, act quickly. Call the emergency medical system (EMS) in the event of severe problems or breathing problems accompanied by chest pain (which may be a sign of heart attack). In every case, check the person's vital signs: heart and breathing rates.

Don't hesitate when it comes to getting help. You should assume that the condition is going to get worse.

If a person is conscious and breathing, you can let him or her get into a comfortable position. Assume a reassuring and calming attitude because panic and stress can make a victim's breathing problems worse. Loosen any tight clothing.

Don't try to prop up the person's head with a pillow. This will close the airway and make it more difficult to breathe. Also, don't try to get the person to eat or drink anything. This could cause choking.

If a person is unconscious and breathing, roll the person into the recovery position — that is, on one side with the top leg and arm bent for support. In the case of a suspected spinal cord injury, don't move the victim unless absolutely necessary.

As you wait for help to arrive, keep track of heart and breathing rates. If the person stops breathing, it's time for artificial respiration (see the next section for how-tos).

Respiratory Arrest and Artificial Respiration

Artificial respiration, sometimes called mouth-to-mouth resuscitation, can be lifesaving when breathing has stopped. It's best performed by someone who has taken a course and is trained in first aid. If you're not sure what you're doing, call EMS right away.

Even when you know how to give artificial respiration, have someone call EMS right away while you begin the technique. If you're alone with a victim, give artificial respiration for a minute or two, quickly make the call yourself and then continue first aid.

To perform artificial respiration, place the person on his or her back. Tilt the head back and lean close to see if the person is breathing. Don't poke around in the person's mouth for a trapped object — you could end up pushing it farther in.

Then, with the person's head tilted back, pinch the nose shut and place your mouth around the victim's. Give two full breaths into the mouth. Each breath should last about one second. You can tell the breath is reaching the lungs if the chest rises and falls with each breath. Let the chest fall before you give the next breath.

All choked up

If the person's chest doesn't rise or fall, chances are the airway is blocked. Tilt the head back farther and try again. If you still don't get results, you'll need to give abdominal thrusts, which are sort of a horizontal version of the Heimlich.

To give abdominal thrusts, straddle the person's thighs. Place the heel of your hand between the navel and the lower tip of the breastbone. Cover it with your other hand and give six to ten quick thrusts straight upward and inward. (Illustrations can be found in Chapter 15.)

Then check to see if the object has been dislodged. To do this, do a "sweep" of the mouth: Hold the tongue and jaw with one hand and slide the index finger of the other hand down the inside of the cheek to the base of the tongue. If the object is there, push it out.

If after this the object is still in the airway, try to give two breaths again with artificial resuscitation. If there's no result, give another six to ten chest thrusts. Continue this cycle until the object is freed or EMS arrives. If the person begins to have seizures, follow the instructions in Chapter 19 for treating them.

For adults — if the heart is still beating — you should give one breath once every five seconds. For infants under 1 year old, give a short puff every three seconds. Children up to age 8 should get a breath every four seconds.

As long as the person is not breathing, keep giving breaths. You should continue until the person begins breathing again or until EMS arrives.

If the person's heart stops, you'll need to provide cardiopulmonary resuscitation (CPR), a combination of artificial respiration and chest thrusts. See Chapter 19 for a description of CPR.

Altitude Sickness

At sea level, the air is compressed by the weight of the rest of the atmosphere bearing down upon it. But at heights of as little as 10,000 feet (Mt. Everest is measured at 29,028 feet), the air is thinner and contains less oxygen, which makes it harder to breathe. At 18,000 feet, in fact, you'll get only half as much oxygen per breath as you would at sea level. This lack of oxygen throws the body out of whack, which may cause temporary illness. In severe cases, it may even cause death.

Symptoms

The symptoms of altitude sickness include

- ✔ Difficulty breathing
- ✔ Difficulty sleeping
- ✔ Decline of physical abilities
- ✔ Confusion or mental sluggishness

Some people describe altitude sickness as something like a hangover — tiredness, fatigue, and nausea.

First to Last

If you're just touring the mountains for a day or two by car, altitude sickness probably won't be much of a concern. But the longer you stay up high, and the more you exert yourself, the more of a concern this condition may be.

To prevent altitude sickness, take it slow. If you're planning a climb or hike at a high altitude, rest up a few days before you head up there. And If possible, come back down to below 2,000 feet before you go to sleep. Experts say "sleeping low" is one of the keys to preventing altitude sickness.

If sickness occurs, take it seriously. Don't climb any higher until your symptoms go away. If they persist for more than a day or two, descend to a lower altitude and again, take it easy. Seek medical attention if your condition worsens.

Severe altitude sickness may lead to high-altitude pulmonary edema (or HAPE), a life-threatening condition in which fluid collects in the lungs. HAPE is marked by headache, nausea, hallucinations, shortness of breath, coughing up blood, and a gurgling sound in the chest. If untreated, it eventually means coma and possibly death.

Asthma

Of course, not every breathing problem involves respiratory failure. Asthma, for example, is a recurring disease caused by inflammation in the lungs. When an attack occurs, the passages within the lungs become narrow and interfere with breathing. A person is able to breathe in but unable to breathe out, and carbon dioxide builds up in the system.

What triggers an asthma attack? It could be cold weather, allergies, stress, or a vigorous workout, among other things.

Symptoms

Signs of an asthma attack include

- Coughing and wheezing
- Tightness in the chest
- Nostrils flaring with each breath

In a severe attack, a person may experience

- An inability to speak
- Blue skin and fingernails
- Increased heart rate
- Perspiration
- Anxiety

First to last

People who've been diagnosed with the condition usually have been prescribed an inhaler or other medicine to stop the attack. Help the person into a comfortable position and help him or her take the medicine. If the person doesn't have medicine or doesn't improve, seek medical attention right away. Remain calm — and do your best to keep the victim calm — during an attack. Panic just makes it more difficult to catch your breath.

If you spot an asthma attack coming on, a remedy might keep it from getting worse. Suggestions from the natural first-aid kit include the herbs ephedra (which can be eaten raw or brewed into a tea), cayenne and lobelia (which can be steeped in alcohol and water to create a tincture), and *Arsenicum,* a homeopathic remedy that soothes anxiety and restlessness. Don't, however, rely on natural remedies if the problem is anything other than mild.

If asthma hasn't been previously diagnosed, write down any symptoms that occur and seek medical attention so the problem can be correctly identified. Other conditions may cause breathlessness — for example, the primary symptoms of congestive heart failure are wheezing and difficulty breathing. It's worth a trip to the doc to ensure proper care.

Croup

This condition is a viral infection that usually occurs in children. With croup, the larynx (voicebox) and trachea (windpipe) become swollen, which narrows the airway and makes breathing noisy and difficult The infection also produces a lot of mucus, which collects in the child's throat and interferes with breathing. Croup often kicks in after a cold, and it's most common between October and March. Most cases aren't dangerous — though they may give a parent a scare.

Symptoms

Croup is marked by

- A whistling sort of wheezing
- A sharp bark, like the bark of a seal
- Difficulty breathing
- Dizziness
- Numb fingers and toes
- Confusion and restlessness
- Hoarseness

First to last

Croup usually disappears on its own in less than seven days. While it's flaring up, however, there are some steps you can take.

First, keep the child calm. If he or she relaxes, the airways will relax and widen, too.

You can also use steam to soften mucus in the airways and make breathing easier. Take the child into the bathroom and close the door. Then turn the shower and sinks on to hot and fill the room with steam. About 15 minutes in the steamy room should do it. Alternatively, use a cool water humidifier in the child's room to help loosen mucus.

To give a steam bath extra croup-relieving power, add about a dozen drops of eucalyptus oil to the humidifier or water source. Homeopathic remedies include *Aconite* and *Spongia,* which are thought not only to relieve coughing but relax a restless child.

Another tactic is to take the child outside on a cool night. Breathing the cool air will also loosen up air passages.

Most bouts of croup pass within a few hours. A pediatrician may recommend decongestants or cortisone medications to loosen the airways and reduce swelling. However, cough syrups aren't a good idea because they don't fight the infection and actually interfere with the child's ability to cough up the mucus in the throat.

If croup doesn't improve in a week or the child begins drooling, hanging the head, sticking out the jaw when breathing, or develops a fever, seek medical attention. These are symptoms of *epiglottitis,* an inflammation of the back of the throat. Epiglottitis can block breathing and should be treated as soon as possible. In the meantime, keep the child in a sitting position to help make breathing easier.

Hyperventilation

There is such a thing as breathing too quickly, and it's called hyperventilation. Usually associated with stress and anxiety, hyperventilation can also be brought on by certain medical conditions and even medications. Hyperventilation is also a symptom of some conditions. For example, if a child breathes rapidly, it's possible he or she is coming down with a fever.

Symptoms

Hyperventilation is marked by rapid, shallow breathing. Other symptoms that may accompany hyperventilation include

- Anxiety
- Rapid heart beat
- Tightness in the throat
- Numbness in the hands, arms, or legs
- Lightheadedness
- Sweaty or cramped hands

What's the danger of breathing too rapidly? The balance of oxygen and carbon dioxide in the blood is thrown off, which causes dizziness and unconsciousness.

Asthma, thyroid problems, and other conditions are associated with hyperventilation, so if this problem happens more than once, visit a doctor for an official diagnosis. *Remember:* you can't handle a problem correctly until it's been correctly identified.

First to last

If someone is breathing too quickly, remain calm and reassuring. Have the person consciously try to take slower, deeper breaths. Breathing into a paper bag can help the person get back into a normal breathing pattern. If a bag isn't handy, cover the mouth loosely with a clean towel or just use the hands. Stick with this technique until breathing slows.

If the person faints, don't panic. In the case of hyperventilation, normal breathing should resume once the person becomes unconscious. If that's the case, you don't need to seek medical care unless the person experiences another attack. Just treat the person for unconsciousness, which is described in Chapter 19.

Chapter 19

Sudden Illness, Swift Response

In This Chapter

▶ Handling heart attack

▶ Recognizing stroke

▶ Understanding seizures and epilepsy

▶ Getting help for unconsciousness and fainting

▶ Taking care of diabetic emergencies

▶ Preventing and giving care for anaphylactic shock

*H*eart disease, epilepsy, diabetes. These are just a few of the long-term conditions that may turn into sudden illnesses that call for first aid. Heart disease, for example, can trigger a heart attack. And a person with diabetes may require emergency care if blood sugar levels get too high or too low. This chapter deals with such sudden problems that might arise from an existing medical condition — those that might just come out of the blue.

Heart Attack

Although a heart attack, also called *myocardial infarction* in medical circles, comes on suddenly, it can be brought about by a condition called *coronary heart disease (CHD)*. With CHD, fatty deposits build up on the walls of the arteries that feed the muscle of the heart. Other times, a clot or other blockage in those arteries can cause a heart attack. When deposits or clots completely block those arteries, the muscle can't get the blood and oxygen it needs and the heart can become damaged. The interruption of oxygen to the cells is called a heart attack.

The danger of a heart attack is this: If the heart muscle becomes damaged, it can't pump blood effectively throughout the rest of the body. In fact, the heart may stop altogether, which can be fatal.

A heart attack is a scary thing because it can happen so quickly. Some people may know they have coronary heart disease and that they're at risk, but others don't expect a thing until a heart attack strikes.

Who's at risk? Well, heart attack is usually associated with older adults, smokers, people with heart disease in their families, those who eat a diet high in fat and cholesterol, and people with diabetes or high blood pressure.

Symptoms

The symptoms of a heart attack can be confused with indigestion and other minor chest pains. So how do you know what the real deal is? Here are some clues:

- A feeling of pressure, fullness, squeezing or pain in the chest. The pain lasts more than a few minutes or goes away and then comes back.
- Pain in the shoulders, neck, or jaw that runs down the arms or back
- Dizziness
- Fainting
- Sweating
- Nausea
- Weakness with minimal exercise (such as climbing stairs)
- Clammy skin and sweating
- Blue skin or lips
- Chest pain during exertion or stress that subsides during a period of rest
- Indigestion that antacids cannot relieve
- Irregular heartbeat
- Difficulty breathing
- Shock
- Unconsciousness

To complicate diagnosis, not all of these warning signs accompany every heart attack. A good rule of thumb is this: If you suspect a heart attack, call on the emergency medical system (EMS) immediately. Even people who seem unlikely candidates for heart attack can suffer them without warning, so it's better to be safe than sorry.

First to last

A heart attack is one of those emergencies in which every second counts, so call EMS immediately if one occurs. The better the care provided in the first two hours after the attack sets in, the greater the chance for survival and recovery.

While you're waiting for EMS to arrive, remain calm and reassuring and try to make the victim comfortable. Loosen any tight clothing, and cover the person up with a blanket. The person can lie down or sit up — in fact, he or she may find it easier to breathe while sitting up.

Next, help the person take any medication he or she may have for the condition. If the person has been diagnosed with heart disease, he or she may have been prescribed nitroglycerin, a pill that's dissolved under the tongue, to take in the event of chest pain. If the attack is a case of temporary chest pain (called *angina*), the nitroglycerin should work within three minutes. If chest pain continues, get medical help right away. Don't give any food or drink to the victim.

Of course, you must keep an eye on vital signs — heart rate and breathing rate — while providing first aid. If the person stops breathing or the heart stops, begin cardiopulmonary resuscitation (CPR) immediately (if you've been trained to do so).

Cardiopulmonary resuscitation: Knowing CPR for life

Cardiopulmonary resuscitation is a combination of artificial respiration (sometimes called mouth-to-mouth resuscitation) and chest compressions, which puts pressure on the heart and forces blood through the circulatory system. It's for more than just heart attack victims. In fact, it should be used in any emergency when a person's heart stops.

Aspirin: Not just for headaches anymore

When signs of a heart attack appear, the first thing you should do is reach for the phone and call for emergency help. Then, says the American Heart Association (and many other experts), reach for the medicine cabinet for that aspirin.

Aspirin, given when chest pain or other heart attack symptoms appear, reduces the risk of death from a heart attack. The medication helps to thin the blood, which allows it to flow through any narrowed blood vessels more easily. And taken on a regular basis as a preventive measure, aspirin may help prevent blood clots that cause attacks and stroke in the first place.

Suggested first-aid dosage is 325 milligrams. If the aspirin has a coating, it must be crushed or chewed for quick results.

A 50 to 100 milligrams-a-day aspirin habit is recommended for people who have been diagnosed with heart disease or have already had a heart attack or a stroke (discussed in the next section) — unless a doctor says otherwise. If you're healthy, however, the Food and Drug Administration says there's no reason for such a regimen. Speak to your practitioner before taking aspirin regularly.

CPR is best performed by someone who has taken a course and is trained in first aid. Instructions are provided below, but if you haven't been trained or are not sure what you're doing, call EMS right away. Even when you know how to give artificial respiration, have someone call EMS right away while you begin the technique.

CPR for adults

Here are the steps you should take for adults. You should follow these if you have been properly trained to do so.

1. **See if the person is conscious. Ask loudly, "Are you OK?" to see if you get a response.**

2. **Call for help. Ask a bystander to call EMS.**

3. **Lay the person on the back. Use the log-roll technique and move the whole person as a unit to minimize injury.**

4. **See if the person is breathing.**

   Tilt the head back and lift up the person's chin. (See Step 1 in Figure 19-1.) Then lean close to the mouth and listen and feel for a breath. (See Step 2 in Figure 19-1).

5. **If the person isn't breathing, give artificial respiration.**

   Pinch the nose shut and place your mouth around the victim's. Give two full breaths into the mouth. (SeeStep 3 in Figure 19-1.) Each breath should last about 1 second. You can tell the breath is going into the lungs if the chest rises and falls with each breath. Let the chest fall before you give the next breath.

6. **After you've given the breaths, check the person's pulse.**

   (See Step 4 in Figure 19-1.) To take a pulse, place the middle and index fingers against the carotid artery in the neck between the voice box at the front of the throat and the muscle at the side of the neck, under the ear. There's a carotid artery on either side of the neck.

7. **If you can't find a pulse, get ready to begin chest compressions.**

   With one hand, feel for a notch at the lower end of the breastbone and measure two finger widths above that notch. (See Step 5 in Figure 19-1.) Place the heel of the other hand at that spot on the breastbone. Cover that hand with the other and interlock the fingers. Don't put your fingers against the chest — just the heel of the hands.

8. **Once the hands are in place, lock your elbows and position your body directly over your hands. (See Step 6 in Figure 19-1.) Give 15 chest compressions in 10 seconds, depressing the breastbone 1½ to 2 inches with each thrust.**

9. **After 15 compressions, give the person two full breaths with artificial respiration.**

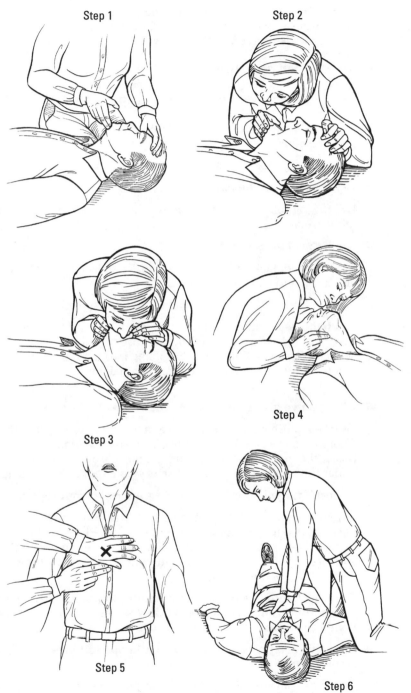

Step 1

Step 2

Step 3

Step 4

Step 5

Step 6

Figure 19-1: These six illustrations demostrate how to perform CPR on an adult.

10. **Check the pulse again. If there is no pulse, repeat the 15 compressions. Continue with this cycle of 2 breaths and 15 compressions until the person is revived or EMS arrives.**

CPR for children ages 1 to 8

Here are the steps to perform CPR on children 1 to 8 years old:

1. **See if the child is conscious. Ask loudly, "Are you OK?" to see if you get a response.**

2. **Call for help. Ask a bystander to call EMS.**

3. **Lay the child on the back.**

   Use the log-roll technique and move the whole child as a unit to minimize injury.

4. **See if the child is breathing.**

   Tilt the head back and lift up the chin. Then lean close to the mouth and listen and feel for a breath.

5. **If the child isn't breathing, give artificial respiration.**

   Pinch the nose shut and place your mouth around the victim's. Give two full breaths into the mouth. Each breath should last about 1 second. You can tell the breath is going into the lungs if the chest rises and falls with each breath. Let the chest fall before you give the next breath.

6. **After you've given the breaths, check the child's pulse.**

   To take a pulse, place the middle and index fingers against the carotid artery in the neck. It can be found in the indentation between the voice box at the front of the throat and the muscle at the side of the neck, under the ear. There's a carotid artery on either side of the neck.

7. **If there's no pulse, get ready to begin chest compressions.**

   With one hand, feel for a notch at the lower end of the breastbone and measure two finger widths above that notch. Place the heel of the other hand at that spot on the breastbone. Cover that hand with the other and interlock the fingers. Don't put your fingers against the chest — just the heel of the hands.

8. **Once the hands are in place, lock your elbows and lean over your hands. Give 5 chest compressions in 4 seconds, depressing the breastbone 1 to 1½ inches with each thrust.**

9. **After five compressions, give the child one full breath with artificial respiration.**

10. **Check the pulse again. If there is no pulse, repeat the five compressions. Continue with this cycle of one breath and five compressions until the child is revived or EMS arrives.**

New and improved CPR?

Cardiopulmonary resuscitation (CPR) as we know it has been the gold standard of first aid for decades. Yet researchers are working on a new way to deliver the heart-helping technique: Instead of using your hands, they say, try this new gadget instead.

The gadget is a hand-held suction device — something like a plunger. When used to compress the chest of a heart attack victim, it's able to push blood through the body's systems more forcefully, helping organs and tissues get the nutrients they need to survive. A study published by the *New England Journal of Medicine* in 1999 found patients who underwent the "plunger method" — officially called active compression-decompression resuscitation — were more likely to come through without brain damage and were more likely to live for more than a year.

While it's available in Europe, the device has yet to be approved by the Food and Drug Administration in the United States. But look out! It may be coming soon to a hospital or paramedic unit near you.

CPR for infants under 1 year

Here are the steps to perform for infants under 1 year old:

1. **See if the infant is conscious by gently shaking the baby's shoulder.**

2. **Call for help. Ask a bystander to call EMS.**

3. **Lay the infant on the back.**

   Use the log-roll technique and move the whole infant as a unit to minimize injury.

4. **See if the infant is breathing.**

   Tilt the head back and lift up the infant's chin. (See Step 1 in Figure 19-2.) Then lean close to the mouth and listen and feel for a breath. (See Step 2 in Figure 19-2.)

5. **If the infant isn't breathing, give artificial respiration.**

   Place your mouth around the victim's nose and mouth. (See Step 3 in Figure 19-2.) Give two full breaths. Each breath should last about 1 second. You can tell the breath is going into the lungs if the chest rises and falls with each breath. Let the chest fall before you give the next breath.

6. **After you've given the breaths, check the baby's pulse.**

   To take a pulse in an infant, check the brachial artery in the arm. Gently press two fingers on the inside of the arm, between the elbow and the shoulder and feel for 5 to 10 seconds. (See Step 4 in Figure 19-2.)

Step 1

Step 2

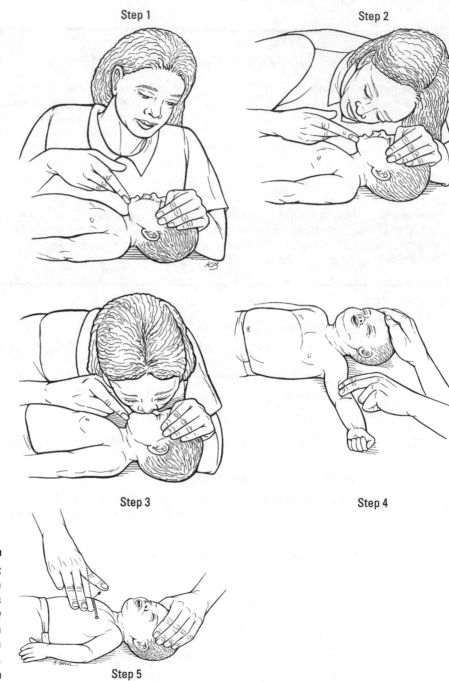

Step 3

Step 4

Figure 19-2:
These five
illustrations
show how
to perform
CPR on an
infant.

Step 5

Transient ischemic attacks, or ministrokes

Not every stroke is a full-blown brain attack. Ministrokes, medically called *transient ischemic attacks, or TIAs*, occur when blood flow to the brain is only briefly blocked, causing symptoms that subside within 24 hours.

Ministroke symptoms are very similar to stroke symptoms. They include temporary weakness, clumsiness or loss of feeling in an arm, leg or side of the face, particularly on one side of the body; temporary dimness or loss of vision; temporary loss of speech or difficulty in communicating; or loss of consciousness.

Ministrokes are a medical red alert. Just like thunder signals a downpour is on the way, a TIA is strong indication that stroke may strike. In fact, a person who has a TIA is nearly ten times more likely to have a stroke than someone of the same age and sex who hasn't had one. Victims should take a ministroke as a warning of a high risk of stroke and enable their doctors to find and treat whatever underlying problems can be treated.

7. **If there's no pulse, get ready to begin chest compressions.**

   Keeping the head back, locate the breastbone, just below the level of the nipples. Hold that spot with an index finger, then place the next two fingers lower down on the breastbone. Lift the index finger and use those two middle fingers for compression.

8. **With your elbow bent, use those middle fingers to give compressions. Give five compressions in 3 seconds, depressing the breastbone ½ to 1 inch each time. (See Step 5 in Figure 19-2.)**

9. **After five compressions, give the infant one full breath with artificial respiration.**

10. **Check the pulse again. If there is no pulse, repeat the five compressions. Continue with this cycle of one breath and five compressions until the infant is revived or EMS arrives.**

Stroke

It's already been said that a heart attack is caused by a lack of blood flow to the heart. A stroke is essentially the same thing, except that it occurs in the brain. With stroke, an artery providing blood to the brain becomes blocked or bursts and the tissues of the brain can't receive the oxygen and nutrients they need to survive. It's because of this similarity that stroke is also sometimes called a *brain attack*.

Fever and seizures

Kids who have high fevers — that is, a temperature above 99 degrees F — sometimes suffer febrile seizures even if they're not seriously ill. These seizures, which occur when body temperature changes rapidly, give parents a scare but usually aren't dangerous and resolve on their own.

If a seizure occurs, try to bring the child's temperature back down to normal with a cool sponge bath or a fan. Don't, however, put the child into a bathtub; if another seizure occurs, the child could choke on the water. Also talk to the child's doctor about the seizure, its cause, and ways to bring temperature down.

Because brain tissue is damaged with each passing moment when it's deprived of oxygen, fast action is necessary with stroke first aid.

Symptoms

Some signs of stroke include

- ✔ Dizziness and falling
- ✔ Slurred speech or loss of speech
- ✔ Sudden, severe headache
- ✔ Weakness or numbness in a part of the body, particularly the face or arm or leg of one side of the body
- ✔ Blurred vision or loss of vision, particularly in one eye
- ✔ Unconsciousness

First to last

If you find yourself with a person who's having a stroke, check breathing and heart rate. If either stop, begin CPR if you are trained to do so. Have a bystander call EMS as soon as possible. The faster a person gets to the hospital, the sooner he or she can receive "clot-busting" medications or surgery to help restore blood flow — techniques that reduce the risk of permanent brain damage. So act quickly. Minutes matter.

If the person is stable, have him or her rest until EMS arrives. Don't try to give any food, water, or medications, and keep a close eye on vital signs. Make the person comfortable, loosening any tight clothing.

Sometimes a person having a stroke will become unconscious. If this happens, get the person into the recovery position — on one side with the upper arm and leg bent to support the body. Stay with the person until medical help arrives.

Seizures and Epilepsy

You may not realize it, but your brain is a hotbed of electrical activity. Inside your noggin, tiny sparks of energy are stimulating millions of cells each time you think a thought or move a muscle.

Seizures, brief periods of involuntary muscle movement, occur when the electricity in the brain becomes uncontrolled. Cells are abnormally stimulated, causing twitching and jerking muscles, drooling, and other symptoms. A single seizure usually lasts 30 to 45 seconds.

Conditions associated with seizures include high blood pressure, brain injuries (such as stroke) and brain illnesses (such as cancer), fever in children, electric shock, poisoning, choking, and drug and alcohol overdose or withdrawal.

When seizures recur without reason, the condition is called *epilepsy,* or *seizure disorder*. Fortunately, epilepsy can usually be controlled with medications.

Symptoms

A seizure may have the following characteristics:

- ✔ Short period of confusion or unconsciousness
- ✔ Tingling or twitching in a part of the body
- ✔ Rigid muscles or jerking muscle movements
- ✔ Grunting or snorting
- ✔ Drooling or frothing at the mouth
- ✔ Loss of bowel or bladder control
- ✔ Loss of consciousness
- ✔ Blue discoloration of the lips, due to temporary cessation of breathing

A brief period of confusion or blackout is called a *petit mal seizure*. A seizure that involves jerking, twitching, rigid muscles, and spasms is termed a *grand mal* seizure

People who've had seizures before can sometimes feel when one is coming on. Signs include a funny taste in the mouth, hallucinations, abdominal pain, or just a feeling that something is going to happen.

First to last

Once a seizure begins, it cannot be stopped. But you can keep the person from injury and call for medical help if necessary.

You should call EMS if the person has more than one seizure an hour or seizures that last longer than two minutes. Also call if the person doesn't wake up between seizures. Emergency care is also necessary for people who've never had a seizure before, people with high blood pressure, and pregnant women. People who have a seizure in water or who are otherwise ill or injured should also get EMS attention.

If an infant experiences seizures for the first time, assume the reason is poisoning. Call the poison control center immediately, and check out Chapter 12.

If the person feels a seizure coming on, help the person lie on the ground to prevent a fall. Loosen the person's clothing and clear the area of any hard objects the person might run into. If pillows are available, place them around to cushion the victim. Don't move the victim unless there's a danger that can't be moved (such as a flight of stairs he or she might topple down).

While a seizure is occurring, don't try to hold the person down and don't put anything in the mouth or between the person's teeth (such as a spoon or a pencil) during a seizure. The person won't be able to stop the seizure, so just wait until it runs its course and do your best to protect the victim from injury.

If the person stops breathing and becomes blue in the face, don't (yes — you read that right) try to give artificial respiration. The seizure will end and the person will begin breathing again before brain damage can occur.

After the seizure has ended, move the person into the recovery position — on one side with the upper arm and leg bent for support. This position will help any fluids drain from the mouth and nose. Don't try to give the person any food or fluids until he or she is fully recovered.

It helps to know that people who have a history of seizures usually experience a specific recovery cycle. Most people wake up for a short time after the seizure has passed and then go into a deep sleep. The person will wake up later feeling disoriented and confused, but will gradually begin to remember where he or she is and what happened.

As a person recovers from a seizure, keep an eye on vital signs. Stay with the person until he or she recovers or medical help arrives.

Unconsciousness

Unconsciousness is not a condition, per se. Rather, it is a state in which a person is unresponsive to surroundings. Fainting is a form of unconsciousness that is brief. Long-term unconsciousness may be deemed a coma.

The person may appear to be asleep, but can't be woken up. An unconscious person also can't clear the throat, cough, or turn the head to one side. This means unconscious victims are at risk of choking.

What causes unconsciousness? Pretty much any medical condition or injury can do it, from a hit on the head to a heart attack.

If you come across someone who's unconscious, look for a Medic Alert tag that may give you a clue about the victim's condition. Along with aid for unconsciousness, provide care for that problem.

A person may slip in and out of consciousness and be incoherent and disoriented. A victim who is deeply unconscious will be motionless and won't speak.

First to last

When someone's unconscious, first look to see if you can quickly determine what happened. Check for obvious injuries or a Medic Alert tag for clues. Call EMS if there's a discernible reason for unconsciousness, give first aid for that particular injury.

If you don't know why a person is unconscious, start by checking the vital signs — heart rate and breathing rate. If a person's heart or breathing has stopped, begin CPR if you are trained to do so.

If you're sure that a person doesn't have a spinal cord injury, get him or her into the recovery position — on one side with the top leg and arm bent for support. This position opens up the airway and reduces the risk of choking, which is the main concern with an unconscious person.

A few caveats with unconsciousness: Because of the risk of choking, don't give the person any food or drink while he or she is unconscious. For the same reason, don't prop his or her head up with a pillow — this angle just makes it harder to breathe. You also shouldn't try to wake an unconscious person by spraying water on the face or slapping the person. The person should be allowed to wake naturally.

Seizures, discussed earlier in this chapter, may occur in an unconscious person. In addition, some people, although they're not having a seizure, become restless and thrash about. If this happens, try to gently restrain the person. However, don't restrain someone who's actually having a seizure.

If a person doesn't revive shortly, call EMS for help. An instance of unconsciousness, even if brief, should be discussed with a physician.

Fainting

Fainting is a brief loss of consciousness — usually so unexpected that the person collapses and falls to the ground. It can be caused by a number of factors, including emotional distress, low blood sugar, or standing in one place for too long.

Symptoms

Symptoms of fainting include

- Pale skin
- Perspiration
- Dizziness
- Nausea
- Unconsciousness

First to last

If you see a person who looks about to faint, act fast. Catch or cushion him or her to keep him or her from falling.

Then lay the person down and elevate the legs about 12 inches from the ground. Use a pile of books, a rolled up blanket, or whatever else you have handy to raise the legs. This position will help blood flow to the brain and restore consciousness. Don't put a pillow under the head because this will make breathing more difficult.

While the person is lying down, check the vital signs — heart and breathing rate — and begin CPR if necessary, and if you are trained. Also, loosen any tight clothing. You might also put a cool cloth on the forehead.

Don't throw water on the person's face or shake or slap the person. If the person vomits, roll him or her into the recovery position — on one side with the top leg and arm bent for support. This position helps protect from choking.

A person who has fainted usually revives quickly. If the victim is unconscious for more than five minutes or is elderly, call EMS.

Diabetic Emergencies

Diabetes is a condition in which a person's cells are somehow unable to use the sugar that's in the bloodstream. As a result, the blood might have too much or too little sugar, which can throw off the way the body functions.

A person with too little sugar in the blood is said to have *hypoglycemia,* which can lead to insulin shock. Too much sugar in the blood is called *hyperglycemia,* and that can mean diabetic coma. Both can be life-threatening if untreated.

A person who is having a diabetic emergency may act drunk or disoriented. A Medic Alert tag is a good clue to what's going on, so check for one.

Symptoms

Symptoms of hypoglycemia, which progresses rapidly, include

- ✔ Hunger
- ✔ Pale skin
- ✔ Disorientation
- ✔ Fast, shallow breathing
- ✔ Seizures in serious cases

Symptoms of hyperglycemia, which progresses gradually, include

- ✔ Thirst
- ✔ Vomiting
- ✔ Flushed skin

> ✔ Frequent need to urinate
>
> ✔ Fast, shallow breathing

The two conditions — though medical opposites — are often hard to differentiate.

First to last

If a person has low blood sugar, have the person eat something sweet, such as a small amount of orange juice, a sugar cube, or a few candies. A sugary snack should restore the person in about 10 minutes. If it doesn't help, seek medical attention right away.

If a person has high blood sugar, seek medical help immediately. The person will need a shot of a medication called insulin to bring blood sugar levels down. If there's insulin on hand, help the person administer it, but still seek professional care.

At times, you won't be able to tell whether a person has high or low blood sugar — and that person might not know either. In that case, give the person a little sugar to see if it helps. If the victim's condition improves, low blood sugar was the culprit. If high blood sugar is the problem, the little bit of extra sugar won't do any harm.

When a victim is unconscious, call EMS right away. Don't prop up the person's head with a pillow (which makes it harder to breathe) and don't give the person anything to eat or drink. An unconscious person is unable to swallow and may inhale the food or liquid and choke.

Anaphylactic Shock

Another kind of sudden illness is *anaphylactic shock,* a condition that's the result of a severe allergic reaction. Few people suffer such strong reactions, but when they do, it's often after contact with bee stings or foods such as peanuts and shellfish.

Though its causes may seem trivial, anaphylactic shock is very serious. In fact, it can result in death in as little as five minutes. You see, the allergic reaction can cause the airways to swell up, cutting off breathing.

Symptoms

Signs of anaphylactic shock include

- Coughing and wheezing
- Difficulty breathing
- Tightness in the chest
- An itchy rash or hives
- Swelling of the face, tongue, and mouth
- Bluish tint to the skin
- Dizziness
- Nausea and vomiting

If you know you have an allergy that causes a serious reaction, you should do two things to protect yourself against anaphylactic shock. First, you should ask your doctor about a prescription for epinephrine, a drug that can stop the reaction and possibly save your life. Then keep the medication on hand at all times. You should also invest in a Medic Alert bracelet so those around you can help if you have a problem.

First to last

If you find yourself with someone having a severe allergic reaction, call EMS right away. Then check the vital signs — breathing and heart rate — and give CPR If necessary, and if you are trained.

The only thing that can stop the reaction is epinephrine. A person known to have strong allergic reactions may carry a dose of the medication along for use in the event of an emergency. If that's the case, help the person use it, following the instructions on the kit. Epinephrine usually comes in a special "autoinjector" syringe in a prepared dose that can be administered quickly and easily.

While waiting for EMS, keep checking vital signs. Help the person into a position where he or she can breathe easily. If the person becomes unconscious, use the recovery position — on one side with the top leg and arm bent for support.

Chapter 20

Muscle, Bone, and Joint Injuries

● ●

In This Chapter

▶ Defining bone and joint injuries

▶ Providing first aid for fractures and dislocations

▶ Applying splints and slings from head to toe

▶ Soothing sprains and strains

● ●

*T*he skeleton is the strong frame of the body. Muscles are flexible bundles of cells that cling to the skeleton and enable you to run, jump, and play and then flop on the couch when you're done.

Even though the muscles and the bones of the body are strong, they can be stretched or broken if a great deal of force is applied — or even if a little bit of force is applied in just the right way, at the right angle. For example, change directions suddenly when you're playing tennis, and you may sprain your ankle. Trip and fall at an awkward angle, and you could be looking at a fractured wrist. Run up against the steering wheel during a car accident, and you could suffer a broken rib.

This chapter is all about bone and muscle injuries and how to handle them.

What's What: The Difference Between Bone and Muscle Injuries

Before you whip out the slings and bandages, here's some background on the main types of bone and muscle injuries that occur.

Fractures

A *fracture* is the proper medical term for a broken or cracked bone. In most cases, bones break simply because they're asked to bear more weight than they can handle at a crucial moment. For that reason, participation in sports, falls, and car accidents are common causes of broken bones. Other times, however, bones break easily because they're already weak from diseases such as cancer and osteoporosis.

To get a better grip on the types of fractures that can occur, here's a quick rundown of how doctor's classify these problems:

- ✔ A open fracture is one in which the broken bone is exposed through a wound in the skin. This is also called a compound fracture. See Figure 20-1 for an example of an open and closed fracture.

- ✔ A closed fracture is a simple break in which the bone doesn't pierce the skin. This is also called a simple fracture.

- ✔ A greenstick fracture occurs mostly in the immature long bones (arms and leg bones) of children. In this type of fracture, one side of the bone is fractured, but the other side is unbroken. To imagine a greenstick fracture, picture a branch that's been snapped but is too flexible to break into two pieces.

- ✔ A comminuted fracture is one in which a part of the damaged bone is broken into fragments or shattered.

- ✔ A pathological fracture is one in which the bone was previously weakened by illness or disease — for example, osteoporosis or cancer. Pathological fractures can be of any type: open or closed, greenstick or comminuted.

These five types of fractures can be further classified according to the angle of the break. A transverse fracture occurs at a right angle to the bone — a clean break. An oblique fracture is one in which the bone breaks at a slanting angle.

Signs of a fracture include

- ✔ Pain
- ✔ Swelling
- ✔ Bruising
- ✔ An unusual or misshapen appearance (the bone may look deformed)

In addition, the victim may have heard the bone snap or may be able to move an injured limb in a strange way. The person may also feel the broken bones grinding against each other. X-rays, however, are the most reliable way to diagnose a fracture, especially a closed fracture.

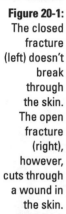

Figure 20-1:
The closed
fracture
(left) doesn't
break
through
the skin.
The open
fracture
(right),
however,
cuts through
a wound in
the skin.

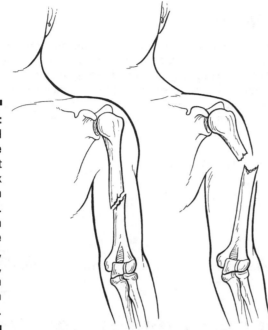

If a child has an accident, suspect a fracture if the child doesn't use the injured limb within a few hours, or if the area remains painful to the touch.

Dislocation

Ever heard the phrase "throw out of joint"? Well, that's the literal definition of dislocation. More specifically, dislocation occurs when a joint is injured in such a way that the bone is displaced. The elbows, fingers, and shoulders are the most at risk for dislocation, which usually occurs because of a fall or blow.

Signs of dislocation include

- ✔ Swelling
- ✔ Unusual, misshapen appearance (the joint may look deformed)
- ✔ Pain
- ✔ Bruising

Dislocation must be treated properly. Without adequate treatment, the joint may not heal properly, making it likely dislocation will occur again in the future.

Strains and sprains

The words sound nearly the same, and they both describe a muscle, ligament, or tendon that's been overworked. There is a subtle difference, however. A strain is an overstretching or minor tearing of a muscle, while a sprain is a significant tear. They're caused by sudden, unaccustomed exercise or a violent blow — like a tackle in football. But sprains and strains don't always seem to happen for a good reason; some occur when you take a wrong step or twist the body in an unusual way.

Symptoms of sprains and strains include

- ✔ Bruising
- ✔ Pain
- ✔ Swelling

X-rays are usually needed to tell a sprain or strain from a fracture.

First Aid for Fractures and Dislocations

Fractures and dislocations are treated the same way — and here's how to do it.

First to last

Regardless of the part of the body involved, basic first aid for fractures and dislocations remains the same. For serious breaks, call (or have someone else call) the emergency medical system (EMS). For more minor injuries, give first aid before seeking medical attention. In both cases, keep an eye on the person's vital signs — heart and breathing rates — and be prepared to give cardiopulmonary resuscitation (CPR) if heart and breathing rates should fail (and if you are trained).

If you've called EMS for assistance, don't move the person in the meantime — emergency personnel know the best way to transport an injured person. If you plan to seek medical attention on your own, make sure the injury is stabilized before carefully moving the person. You can find guidelines for emergency transport in Chapter 7.

The key to first aid for fractures and dislocations is to protect the area against further injury and immobilize it to keep more damage from occurring. One of the best ways to do this is with a splint, a combination of a bandage and rigid materials that holds the injury in place. A sling, a hammock of fabric that supports the area and keeps the pressure off, is another technique. Descriptions of the right splints and slings for specific injuries are coming up in a minute.

First, however, here are some guidelines for open fractures — those breaks in which the bone breaks through the skin:

✔ When handling an open fracture, first remove clothing from the area of the wound. As you would with any bleeding wound, apply pressure to the area using a sterile cloth or bandage. Once bleeding has stopped, gently place a large dressing over the entire wound to cover it and protect it. (See Chapter 5 for details on treating wounds.)

✔ With an open fracture, disturb the wound as little as possible. Don't touch any bone fragments or try to put them back into place, and don't force the bone back into place under the skin. In fact, keep your fingers out of the wound; touching it may cause further injury and contaminate the area with germs.

✔ Once an open fracture is dressed, splint it as you would a closed fracture, taking care to raise the area above the level of the heart. This action should reduce swelling and bleeding. See the section "Slings and splints from head to toe" for the next step.

Slings and splints from head to toe

Different injuries require different splints and slings, and they're arranged here in head-to-toe order.

Collarbone

Collarbones are easily fractured because they're relatively fragile bones with little support behind them. To protect a broken collarbone, apply a sling.

Start with the triangular bandage from your first-aid kit, which should be about 3 feet by 3 feet by 4.5 feet. Spread the bandage over the torso of the victim, with the longest side along his or her good side. Place the injured arm on top of the bandage, with the opposite point of the triangle under the elbow of the injured arm. Take the bottom point and fold it upward over the arm and tie it around the back of the neck to the other, topmost point. Adjust the sling so the hand is elevated a few inches above the elbow. Pin the point at the elbow to the side of the sling to keep the arm in place. Make sure the fingers are exposed to avoid cutting off circulation.

Once the sling is in place, use another bandage to tie the whole thing against the body to prevent movement. Gently wrap a length of narrow bandage around the torso and injured arm and — not too tightly — knot it in place.

Arm

If the upper arm is injured, apply a sling (described above) and then apply another bandage to tie the whole thing against the chest. See Figure 20-2 for an illustration.

Figure 20-2:
First, apply a splint to the injured area. Once the arm is in a splint, fold a bandage around the arm and neck to keep the arm from moving.

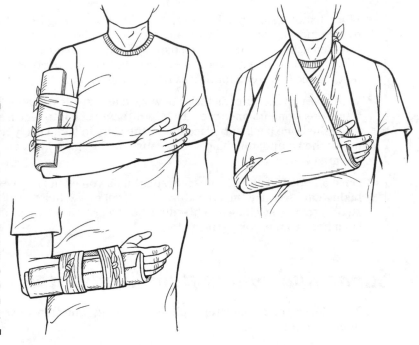

Elbow

A splint is needed to immobilize an injured elbow. If the elbow is in a bent position, splint it in that position. If the elbow is straight, apply the splint to the outside of the arm.

That having been said, how do you apply a splint? First, find a rigid support that will keep the injury in place. Suggestions include sticks, boards, broom handles, cardboard, and even folded-up newspapers and magazines. If the item is rough, wrap it in a towel or blanket to cushion it. Make sure the support is long enough to extend a few inches beyond the injury for maximum stability.

Using first-aid tape, bandages, or makeshift ties (strips of towels, sheets, or even clothing), secure to the injured part of the body. Don't tie any knots near or on top of the injury itself — make your ties above and below that area.

Don't tie the splint too tightly — you may cut off circulation to the injured area, which will cause more harm than good. If the limb begins to tingle or become nunb, loosen the ties on the splint.

Wrist and Hand

To protect an injured wrist or hand, immobilize it by wrapping it with padding. You may use a blanket, a piece of clothing, or even a magazine or newspaper. Then the person's elbow and fashion a sling around the arm.

Finger

Finger injuries don't call for splints or slings. Instead, apply an ice pack wrapped in a towel to reduce pain and swelling and keep the hand elevated. Seek medical attention.

Rib

First aid for a rib injury involves supporting the injured area with a pillow or folded-up blanket. If the person is having trouble breathing, see Chapter 18 on breathing difficulty.

Pelvis

An injured pelvis is a serious matter. Don't move a person when you suspect such an injury has occured — rely on EMS to do that job. If you absolutely must move a person with an injured pelvis, use the clothes drag technique (see Chapther 7).

Hip

As with a pelvic injury, don't move a person with an injured hip unless absolutely necessary. However, if you do need to move the person, you need to apply a really big splint.

Use two boards that have been wrapped in towels. Place one on the outside of the injured hip, stretching from the armpit to the foot. The other board should go along the inside of the leg, from the crotch to the foot. Tie the boards in place around the leg in three places (near the ankle, the knee, and the groin) and then continue to secure the outer board to the torso at chest and waist level.

Leg

If the upper part of the leg has been injured (the bone called the femur), don't move the person unless absolutely necessary. If you must transport a person, apply a splint as you would for a hip injury.

If the lower leg is injured, apply a splint. Find two boards and wrap them in towels to cushion them somewhat. Place one board against the outside of the leg (from hip to foot) and the other against the inside (from crotch to foot). Tie the boards in place around the leg in three places (near the ankle, the knee, and the groin). See Figure 20-3 for an illustration.

What should you do if you don't have anything rigid to use as a splint? With a leg injury, you can secure the injured leg to the uninjured leg — essentially using the good leg for support. If you have a blanket, roll it lengthwise and place it between the legs before you lash the legs together to provide more support.

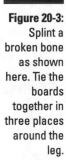

Figure 20-3:
Splint a broken bone as shown here. Tie the boards together in three places around the leg.

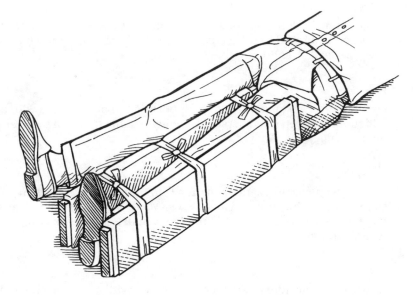

Knee

If the injured knee is already straight, use the same splint you would for an injured leg (described earlier).

For an injured knee that's bent, don't straighten it out! Get the person to bend the good knee to the same angle, and then use that knee as a splint to provide some support. If you have a blanket, roll it up lengthwise and place it between the legs before you tie the legs together to provide more support.

Ankle and foot

An ankle or foot can be immobilized using a pillow or a folded-up towel or blanket. Apply this soft splint by laying the pillow lengthwise underneath the ankle and foot and folding it up and around the joint. Secure it in two places on the lower leg and in another place against the foot (see Figure 20-4). Keep the ankle or foot elevated to help reduce swelling.

Shock: Don't let it happen to you

With practically any injury comes the risk of shock, a failure of the circulatory system to deliver blood and oxygen to the cells that need it. Symptoms of shock include clammy skin, weakness, a bluish tinge to the skin, a faint pulse, and nausea and vomiting. If shock remains untreated, the victim may quickly become unconscious and possibly even die.

To prevent and treat shock, take the following actions:

✔ Place the person in the shock position. This is simply laying the person flat (don't put pillows under the head) and raising the feet about 12 inches. Use books, a blanket, or anything else handy as a support. Don't move the person into the shock position if you suspect a spinal cord injury or if the head, back, neck, or legs have been injured.

✔ Cover the person with a blanket or coat to keep him or her warm.

More on treating shock can be found in Chapter 11.

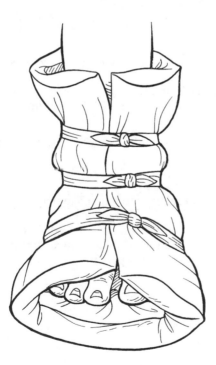

Figure 20-4:
A splint for
an ankle or
a foot.

Toe

An injured toe calls for the application of an ice pack wrapped in a towel to help reduce pain and swelling. Keep the foot elevated, too. You might also want to put some cotton between the toe and its neighbor and tape the two together to immobilize them. If the toe looks deformed, seek medical attention right away.

First Aid for Sprains and Strains

Handling sprains and strains is pretty straightforward. The tricky part is knowing how to tell a sprain from a fracture or dislocation. The truth of the matter is that there is no easy way to tell the difference; unless the injury shows deformities or is an open fracture, an x-ray might be needed to diagnose a sprain. So the moral of the story is this: If you suspect that a fracture or dislocation has occurred, err on the side of caution and seek medical attention.

First to last

If you're sure you're facing a strain or sprain, take the following steps:

- Remove clothing and jewelry from the injured area. If the injury swells with these items still in place, they may restrict blood flow and become impossible to remove.
- Apply an ice pack wrapped in a towel to the area to reduce pain and swelling.
- Elevate the injured area.
- Give an over-the-counter pain reliever to help ease pain.

Remember: It's often hard to tell the difference between different muscle, bone, and joint injuries. If you're in doubt, seek medical attention immediately to make sure the victim is cared for properly.

Part IV
Sports Injuries

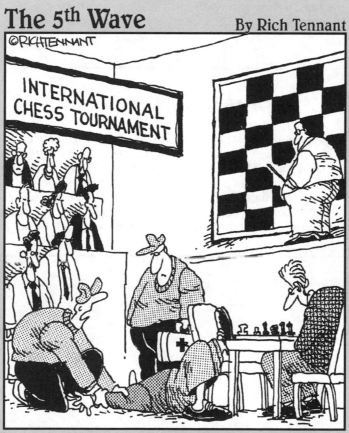

The 5th Wave   By Rich Tennant

INTERNATIONAL CHESS TOURNAMENT

"I'm pretty sure it's just a sprain. He castled pretty hard at the end of that last round."

In this part . . .

*F*ore! You never know what sort of injuries and accidents may happen on the court, the course, or the playing field. This part serves up some of the possibilities and gives you the plays you need to run interference against the most common. Warm up with some tips on prevention and playing it safe, and then touch base on first-aid techniques and teachings you can use on and off the field.

Chapter 21

Preventing Sports Injuries and Accidents

The vote is in! Exercise is good for you. The American College of Sports Medicine and the Centers for Disease Control and Prevention recommend that you get at least 30 minutes of vigorous exercise on most days of the week to reap rewards such as increased energy, a stronger body, and maybe even a slimmer figure. Still, exercise has its downside: an increased risk of injury. The good news is you can minimize that risk by taking a few simple precautions.

Let's Get Started

When you decide to get into shape or play a sport, it's tempting to throw yourself into it wholeheartedly. Think twice, though, about taking that leap before talking with your doctor. Some conditions can be worsened or brought on by exercise, so it's a good idea to get a check-up and an okay from the doc before working out. If you're usually a couch potato, if you have a condition such as heart disease or diabetes, or if you smoke, this advice is especially important. Even when your doc gives you the all-clear, don't give it your all right away. Instead, take it slowly and work up to a level where you feel comfortable. Pushing yourself will only make injuries more likely — and make exercise a chore.

Warm Yourself Up

When it comes to staving off sports injuries, warming up is half the battle. Warming up, or doing a few stretches and easy exercise *before* getting to the main event, gets blood flowing to the muscles you're about to use. This makes them more flexible and less prone to sprains and strains — statistics show that even stretching exercises can reduce the risk of some injuries (particularly leg injuries) by up to 80 percent. Plus, because limber muscles stretch and flex better than cool ones, your performance could even improve thanks to a warm-up.

How do you warm up? Try to choose an activity that involves the same muscles you'll be using when you exercise. If you're going to run, try a brisk walk. If you're going to lift weights, swing your arms around slowly, propeller style. Spend 10 to 15 minutes in whatever activity you choose before moving on to the main event.

Stretch Yourself Out

Once you're warmed up, you need to stretch out. Stretching helps your flexibility, or how far you can move your joints, and it also reduces your risk of injuries such as sprains and strains. Try to hit every muscle when you stretch, including those in the lower back, upper back, chest, shoulders, thighs, lower legs, and arms.

When you stretch, use a smooth motion and don't bounce. For best results, hold the stretch for about 15 seconds. Stretch only as far as is comfortable — you don't want to be in pain!

Do It Right

There's a right way and a wrong way to exercise. If you know the right way, you'll not only be a better player, but you'll be safer, too. The wrong way can lead to sudden injuries or long-term damage.

Think of tennis as one example. If you know the right way to hold the racquet and hit the ball, you're in great shape. But the wrong grip and posture could mean a sore arm or back — and probably a loss on the court. The same goes for weightlifting. Proper form will give your body the advantage when you lift, giving you the ability to progress farther, faster. It also ensures you're working the correct muscles and getting the greatest benefit from your efforts. But using weights improperly could cause a strain or maybe even an accident with the equipment.

Rules and common sense also come into play here. If you're experimenting with a new sport or activity, make sure you know the ropes. Many accidents occur because of ignorance — skating or swimming in an unsafe area, not following signs on ski slopes, or taking a boat out when the weather's turning ominous.

To protect yourself, find someone who knows what they're doing and get a lesson *before* you kick one off or serve one up. Personal trainers and coaches are good sources of information. It may be worth investing in a few lessons from a professional if your sport is something you plan to do regularly.

One more word about equipment: Make sure you have the right stuff before you start getting hot and heavy — and "right stuff" doesn't mean gumption. Instead, it means shoes, clothes (including bras and athletic supporters and cups), eyewear, headgear, mouth guards, weights, sticks, pucks, helmets, pads, nets, clubs, or even polo ponies — anything you might use when you're working out or playing a sport. The wrong equipment, or ill-fitting equipment, can contribute to an injury by not protecting you properly, tripping you up, or rubbing you the wrong way to cause a brush burn or blister.

For information about sporting goods, footwear, and other equipment, again, coaches and trainers are your best bet. Another option is the staffer at your sporting goods store, especially if it's a specialty store focusing on one sport or item.

Know Thy Limits

Exercise was once associated with the phrase, "No pain, no gain." But now, experts are dismissing that idiom as dangerous. Current advice says you should listen to your body while you're exercising or on the playing field. If your knees or arms start sending you signals that they'd like to take a break, listen to them. If you're thirsty, stop and get a drink. Fact is, you're already dehydrated when you feel thirsty. So be sure to drink before, during, and after your workout.

Too much exercise when your body's not used to it can leave you painfully sore the next day or, even worse, can strain or sprain a muscle. And, if you're too tired, your body won't be able to react as well when playing a sport, which leaves you open for trips and falls. You need to watch the temperature, too. If you overexert yourself when it's too hot outside, you may be at risk for heat cramps, heat stroke, or heat exhaustion (see Chapter 17 for more information on these conditions).

Exercise is good for you, but, as they say, moderation in all things.

Finding the zone

When you talk about exercise, you also need to talk about heart rate. For one thing, taxing your heart is dangerous if you're susceptible to high blood pressure, heart disease, and a number of other conditions. For that reason, it's important to follow your doctor's advice if you're in that category.

But even if you're perfectly healthy, it's worth it to pay attention to your heart rate. That's because it plays a part in how fast you metabolize fat — and lose weight. If you're in right zone for your heart rate during exercise, your body will get into a mode where it burns fat easily. But surpass that range, and your body turns to fuel in your bloodstream for energy, leaving the fat where it lies on your thighs.

How do you know what your range is? Experts report you should aim for 70 percent of your maximum heart rate for your age. To determine the maximum rate, subtract your age from 220. Then calculate 70 percent by multiplying the result by 0.7. Keep your pulse per minute close to that figure, and you're right on target for maximum metabolism.

Cool It Down

Once you're done with your game or workout, don't just plop yourself down on the couch. Take a few minutes to cool down — that is, keep moving slowly as your heart and breathing rates get back to normal once you stop exercising. This helps your body adjust its blood flow back to its everyday patterns and prevents problems such as fainting and dizziness, which happen if you call it quits too quickly. As with your warm-up, allow 10 to 15 minutes for this part of the workout.

Of course, even if you're following all the rules, accidents and injuries do happen. The next chapter covers some common problems that may strike — and what you can do about them.

Keep an eye on the kids

Safety on the playground and the playing field is a big issue for kids. To make sure they're safe:

- Make sure kids are supervised at all times.

- Provide equipment that's the right size and in good working order.

- Show kids how to use equipment correctly.

- Keep play relatively calm to avoid accidents "in the heat of the moment."

- Make sure kids are into the game. It's the daydreamer in the outfield who's likely to get hit with the ball.

- Be ready with the first-aid kit.

Chapter 22

First Aid for Sports Injuries and Accidents

- -

In This Chapter

▶ Main types of sports injuries

▶ Why RICE is nice

▶ Common sports injuries and what to do about them

- -

Maybe you're a professional sports star. Or a weekend warrior who thrives on that pick-up game of basketball in the park. Whatever your level of expertise as an athlete, you may want to take a time-out to think about sports injuries and what you'd do if one occurred while you were on the playing field. This chapter addresses that dilemma, giving you information on common injuries and how to take care of them.

The Two Types of Injuries

About 3 to 5 million sports injuries happen every year, and they all fall into one of two categories:

- ✔ *Acute injuries* are those that happen all of a sudden, often in a violent way. They include broken bones and torn ligaments — the sort of traumas that occur from harsh tackles, hard falls, and the like.

- ✔ *Overuse injuries* occur slowly, over time, from repeated stress on a certain part of the body. Running every day for years, for instance, causes wear-and-tear on the legs and knees that may result in an overuse injury. Or overuse might be caused by improper form during play or repeated abnormal motion of a part of the body (such as a golf swing or tennis serve — not something you'd see in nature).

Sports injuries by activity

Based upon information collected by the National Injury Information Clearinghouse and reported to the Consumer Product Safety Commission, the following activities (or their apparel or equipment) were related to the majority of sports injuries in 1997 (latest figures available).

Activity	Number of Injuries
Basketball	644,921
Bicycling	544,561
Football	334,420
Baseball	188,140
Soccer	148,913
Softball	138,574
Snow skiing	No report in 1997
In-line skating	98,414
Trampoline	82,722
Fishing	72,598
Volleyball	67,340
Horseback riding	58,709
Weight lifting	56,724
Roller skating	54,609
Wrestling	39,829
Golf	39,473

Activity	Number of Injuries
Swimming	27,671
Ice skating	25,379
Mountain biking	No report in 1997
Martial arts	24,123
Bowling	23,317
Tennis	22,294
Ice hockey	17,327
Track & field	13,225
Water skiing	10,657
Paddleball/Squash/Racquetball	10,438
Rugby	7,757
Boxing	7,257
Mountain climbing	4,059
Billiards/Pool	3,685
Archery	3,213
Surfing	No report in 1997
Tag sports	No report in 1997

Source: National Electronic Injury Surveillance System, calendar year 1997. Product-associated Visits to Hospital Emergency Rooms Injury Estimates for Calendar Year 1997. U.S. Consumer Product Safety Commission.

RICE, RICE baby

JARGON ALERT

Before you read another word about sport injuries, you need to know all about RICE. This appetizing acronym stands for rest, ice, compression, and elevation, and it describes a first-aid technique used frequently to handle sports injuries. You'll see the word pretty often in this chapter, so learn now what it means.

✔ **R is for rest:** When injury occurs, stop exercising — don't be macho man or superwoman and try to work through the pain. If you keep going, you'll just force more blood into damaged tissue, causing pain and impeding healing.

✔ **I is for ice:** To minimize swelling, apply an ice pack wrapped in a towel to the injured area (see Figure 22-1). Keep the ice in place for about 15 minutes at first, then remove it for 10 minutes, reapply it for 10, remove it for 10, and so on. Do this for the first hour after injury.

✔ **C is for compression:** An elastic bandage wrapped around the injury can keep fluids from accumulating in the injured area. However, don't tie the bandage so tight that blood can't get to that spot. If you cut off circulation, you face the risk of tissue damage and possibly gangrene.

✔ **E is for elevation:** If the injury is to an extremity — like an arm or a leg — raise the injured area above chest level. This position also keeps fluids from accumulating in the injured area.

RICE, keep in mind, is simply a first-aid tactic. An injured athlete should seek medical attention as soon as possible for anything more than a minor injury. And even if the injury is minor, severe pain, swelling, long-term pain (more than two weeks), or discoloration of the injured area are signs you need a doctor's advice.

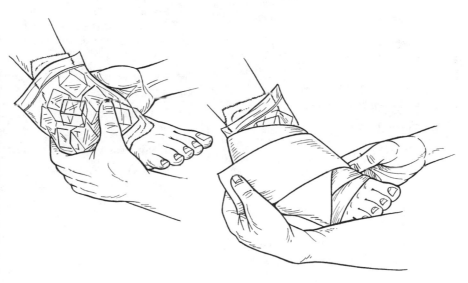

Figure 22-1:
Apply ice to minimize swelling and then wrap an elastic bandage to keep fluids from pooling in the injured area.

When Athletes Are Aching . . .

RICE is great for a host of common sports-related injuries. So what are those injuries? Read on to find out.

Sports and the pains they cause

The following is a list of the injuries you may encounter in various sports. Don't avoid your favorite sport after reading this list; just keep in mind precautions and proper form while you work out.

- **Archery:** Tennis elbow and muscle strains.

- **Badminton:** Rotator cuff injuries, tennis elbow, muscle strains, and plantar fasciitis.

- **Baseball/softball:** Pitcher's elbow, joint sprains, hip pointer, bursitis, shoulder separation, rotator cuff injuries, and jammed finger. Getting hit with a ball may mean broken teeth, a black eye, or a concussion.

- **Basketball/handball/volleyball:** Dislocated or jammed finger, muscle strains, bursitis, rotator cuff injuries, shoulder separation, eye injury, and jumper's leg.

- **Bicycling:** Carpal tunnel syndrome.

- **Football:** Turf toe, shoulder dislocation or separation, hip pointer, and dislocated or jammed finger. Traumatic injuries, such as broken bones, concussion, or black eye, are also common.

- **Golf:** Arthritis, tennis elbow, bursitis, and shoulder separation.

- **Gymnastics:** Stress fracture of wrist, spinal fractures, and heavy calluses. Falls may result in broken bones, torn ligaments, and the like.

- **Hockey:** Stress fractures, Morton's foot pain (caused by too-tight skates), and tailbone pain (from repeated falls on the ice). Most injuries in hockey come from physical contact.

- **Rowing:** Upper and lower back pain.

- **Ice and in-line skating:** Stress fracture, high knee and hip pain, Morton's foot pain, and tailbone pain (from repeated falls).

- **Skiing:** Muscle strains, torn cartilage, torn ligaments, skier's thumb, and altitude sickness. Injuries like broken bones may also occur during falls.

- **Soccer:** Muscle strains, torn cartilage, and torn ligaments.

- **Swimming:** Swimmer's shoulder, swimmer's ear.

- **Tennis:** Tennis elbow, shoulder separation.

- **Running and track and field:** Knee injuries, torn cartilage, sprains and strains, and stress fractures.

Achilles tendon injuries

The Achilles tendon runs from the lower calf to the heel. In flat-footed athletes or those with particularly high arches, the tendon (a tendon attaches a muscle to a bone) can become inflamed. This causes shooting pain during activity, and the tendon may even pop or rupture with too much physical stress.

Mild injuries can be treated with rest and a break from physically stressful activities, such as running. Supportive shoes, stretching, and the application of RICE also help. In severe cases, a cast or physical therapy may be necessary.

Back muscle injuries

The back and spine absorb a lot of the stresses and shocks the body is subjected to, and overuse, twisting and bending, and poor posture can all take their toll. Any imbalance in the way the muscle is used can lead to a back injury. Athletes susceptible to this type of sports-related problem include runners and weightlifters. First aid, again, is RICE, followed by a brief period of rest. However, experts recommend getting up and around as soon as you feel well enough — too much time in bed actually weakens back muscles, putting them at even greater risk of injury.

Blisters

A blister occurs when friction causes a separation between the different layers of the skin, creating a pocket. The painful little pocket then fills with fluid. Blisters are caused most often by poorly fitting shoes and clothing, or repetitive activity that rubs the skin (such as driving a few buckets of golf balls without gloves). First aid is simple: Leave the blister alone. If you wish, you can drain the fluid from the pocket with a sterile needle, but leave the top layer of skin in place as the blister heals.

Blow to the eye

Racquetballs, softballs, and baseballs can all do a great deal of damage with a direct hit on an eye. Signs of injury include cloudy vision, bruising, and blood in the eye itself. First aid for this injury is to cover *both* eyes with a light bandage and get the victim to an eye specialist. Chapter 9 discusses eye injuries in detail.

Broken bone

A sudden fall, a sharp blow, or even an awkward twist can cause a bone to break. Chapter 20, with bone and joint injuries, discusses first aid for a break.

Bursitis

A bursa is a lubricating sac of fluid located within a joint. The bursa, when it's doing its job, lets you move your arm or leg smoothly in its socket. But overuse can cause the bursa to become inflamed — a condition called *bursitis*. Symptoms include pain in the joint during strenuous or repeated motion. First aid includes anti-inflammatory drugs (such as ibuprofen) to lessen the pain. Rest and stretching exercises can help with rehabilitation.

Dislocated finger

Bending or twisting the finger into an awkward position may cause the joint to dislocate, or come out of its socket. With this injury, the tip of the injured finger will point backward, and there may be a lump in the joint itself. Seek medical attention to reset the joint — if it's not done correctly, full function may not be restored. Once the joint is back in place, the fingers can be splinted together for a few days to immobilize them and help the injury heal faster. Gentle exercise is then recommended to keep the joint working as it heals.

Dislocated shoulder

A severe twist or blow to the shoulder can cause dislocation — or the displacement of the arm bone (called humerus) from the joint socket. With a dislocation, the shoulder looks somewhat square, and the arm cannot be lifted out to the side. First aid for dislocation means immobilizing the arm with a sling (details on slings can be found in Chapter 20) and then calling for medical attention. Don't try to "pop" the bone back in yourself, no matter how many times you've seen Mel Gibson do it in *Lethal Weapon*.

Groin pull

A groin pull is a tear in the muscle of the inner thigh. They occur commonly in athletes who change directions quickly while running, run in bursts, or stop and start while running straight ahead. Symptoms include sudden pain in the inner thigh area and possibly bruises that stretch from the crotch to the knee. Immediate first aid is RICE, and activity should be kept to a minimum for about two weeks. Stretching and strength exercises can help rehabilitate the injured area.

Hamstring pulls

A hamstring pull is a tear in the hamstring muscles, which stretch from the base of the buttock down the back of the leg to the knee. They happen among runners and athletes who must propel their legs quickly — for example, basketball players. Treatment includes RICE, followed by rest. In severe cases, crutches may be necessary during recuperation.

Hip pointer

Dive for home plate in baseball (or otherwise fall onto your hip bone), and you may suffer a hip pointer, a bruise to the top of the hip bone. With this injury, the thigh won't move forward. RICE, of course, should be your first step. Then, seek medical attention if pain persists. An athlete should avoid sprints, squat thrusts, and hill running while the injury is healing.

Jammed finger

Catching a ball that's been thrown hard or otherwise putting force on the tip of a finger may cause jammed finger, also called mallet finger. With this condition, the topmost joint of the finger freezes and can't be bent because the tendon has been torn in some way. First aid means RICE and the application of a splint that will keep the finger as straight as possible. Then, seek medical care.

Morton's foot pain

Also called interdigital neuritis, Morton's foot pain is caused by a trapped nerve in the foot. It's characterized by a burning pain between two of the toes, and it feels worse when the foot is squeezed. Foot pads and wider shoes help take the pressure off temporarily, while professional treatment includes cortisone injections and maybe surgery. It occurs in ice skating and hockey when skates are too tight.

Muscle cramps

Cramps are different than sprains or strains in that they don't involve damage or tearing of the muscle. Instead, cramps are caused by muscle fibers suddenly and painfully contracting. They can last a few seconds or several hours. Causes include a salt or mineral deficiency (such as a potassium deficiency), hyperventilation, and a slowing of the blood supply of the muscle. For first aid, encourage the person to stretch and squeeze the affected muscle gently. Eating fruits such as bananas and vegetables can help replace potassium, and a salt deficiency can be corrected by drinking Gatorade or another sports drink.

Nosebleed

Caused most often by trauma, a nosebleed is easy to treat. Have the victim sit upright and pinch the nostrils together for about 5 to 10 minutes until the blood clots. If bleeding doesn't stop, apply an ice pack wrapped in a towel to the bridge of the nose while still holding the nostrils together. Don't tilt the head back to keep blood from running out of the nose — it'll simply flow down the back of the throat into the stomach instead.

Rotator cuff injuries

Skiers, basketball players, golfers, and tennis players — plus other athletes who engage in "throwing" sports — are at risk for rotator cuff injuries. The cuff is the set of muscles that covers the shoulder, rotates the humerus (the upper bone of the arm), and stabilizes the shoulder. Injury occurs with overuse: The cuff muscles rub against the bone and become frayed, which can lead to tear or rupture. Symptoms include pain that occurs when you raise your arms straight out from your sides and up above your head (as if you're flapping your wings). First aid is rest and anti-inflammatory medication. Professional medical treatment may involve steroid injections and physical therapy.

Shin splints

The tibia bone is the front bone in the lower leg, and a shin splint is a tiny tear in the muscle attached to that bone, which causes pain in the front and back parts of the leg. Splints may be caused by an imbalance between the strong back leg muscles and the weaker muscles in the front of the leg. They're also triggered by running on the toes, not stretching properly, and not wearing footwear that absorbs shock well. Treatment includes non-steroidal anti-inflammatory drugs (such as ibuprofen), rest and relaxation, and the purchase of a supportive pair of athletic shoes.

Shoulder separation

The collarbone and the top of the shoulder are held together with ligaments, tough tissues that connect muscles and bones. When these ligaments are torn, the condition is known as separated shoulder. It's marked by pain on the top of the shoulder, and the shoulder may appear misshapen. Moving the arm straight up above the head will also cause pain on top of the shoulder. A sling should be applied to the arm as first aid, then medical treatment should be sought. A number of sports hold the risk for shoulder separation, including baseball, basketball, football, golf, racquetball, tennis, and track and field.

Skier's thumb

Skier's thumb is essentially a sprained thumb — a tearing of the muscle that occurs when the lower thumb joint is wrenched out of place. It's called skier's thumb because it often happens when a skier falls and the strap on the pole forces the thumb in an awkward position. With the injury, the tip of the thumb can move, but the lower joint is swollen and painful, especially when it's moved outward. First aid means RICE, as well as bandaging the joint to keep it in place. A sling for the whole arm will help reduce swelling in the first days after injury.

Sprains and strains

A strain is an overstretching or minor tearing of a muscle, while a sprain is a significant tear. These muscle pulls are likely to occur in the hamstring (the muscle in the back of the thigh) in sprinters; the groin (inner thigh) in basketball players and others who must change direction quickly; the calf in jumpers; and the shoulder in swimmers.

Sprains and strains can be prevented to a degree by stretching, exercising muscles equally, and avoiding ambitious exercise programs. First aid for a minor tear involves applying heat before activity and ice afterward to ease pain. A moderate tear calls for RICE for 20 minutes three to four times a day for about a week. After that period, heat treatments should replace ice. In serious cases, surgery and rehabilitation may be needed.

See Chapter 20 for more on strains and sprains.

Stress fractures

Also called march fractures because they affect soldiers, stress fractures are incomplete cracks in a bone caused by the repeated stress of running or jumping. They occur most often in the shins and the feet.

Symptoms include pain during activity that subsides with rest, a small area that's painful to the touch, and sometimes painful walking. They're caused, among other things, by overdoing it during training, engaging in vigorous aerobics, or jumping with a flat-footed landing.

First aid is basically rest. As fractures heal, which may take several weeks, try a new activity that doesn't put pressure on the area (maybe swimming or bicycling).

Swimmer's ear

Guess what type of athlete suffers from swimmer's ear, a soreness that occurs in the canal of the ear? Chronic wetness and a reaction to salt or chlorine causes this condition. It can also be triggered by overenthusiastic use of cotton swabs. This is a minor condition, but it can be painful. Over-the-counter pain relievers and the application of a warm pad over the ear may ease pain. Also, a doctor may clean out the ear and prescribe drops or a cream to clear up the condition.To keep swimmer's ear from striking, you should dry the ear thoroughly and maybe put a few drops of a preventive alcohol solution (available over the counter) into the canal after swimming.

Swimmer's shoulder

Also called painful arc, shoulder impingement, or subacromial bursa, swimmer's shoulder occurs when the bursa (a lubricating sac found in a joint) becomes trapped between the bone of the arm and the tip of the shoulder. It's caused by overuse of the arm and shoulder and is a risk for competitive swimmers. Usual treatment is rest and over-the-counter pain relievers.

Tendinitis

A tendon is the tissue that attaches a muscle to the bone. Tendinitis is the inflammation of that tissue caused by overuse. In the knees, tendinitis is caused by activity that involves jumping or squatting. In the elbows, it's caused by "throwing" sports like shot-put or javelin toss, as well as pitching. Tendinitis also occurs in the shoulders, brought on by swimming or the rowing involved in canoeing and kayaking. First aid means employing RICE and letting the joint rest. Medical care involves strengthening exercises and possibly steroid injections and physical therapy in serious cases.

Tennis elbow

This condition, a type of tendinitis that occurs most often in tennis players, is the result of constant motions of the forearm as the hand and wrist remain in the same position. The movements inflame the tendons on the outside of the elbow because of the constant irritation of the twisting and rotating. With tennis elbow, pain is felt when the wrist straightens or bends against resistance. Treatment is the application of ice (follow the time intervals in RICE) and rest. Exercises to strengthen the wrist can help with recovery; ask a coach, trainer, or physical therapist for examples of such exercises.

Torn cartilage

Cartilage is the tough, white tissue within a joint that clings to the bone and acts as a shock absorber. In the knee, especially, cartilage may be torn or damaged if a joint is twisted the wrong way. With this injury, symptoms include a tender area between the knee bones. The knee may also be swollen or click or lock when moved. First aid means RICE and supporting the joint with a bandage. Minor tears may heal on their own; others require surgery. Torn cartilage is associated with skiing, soccer, and track and field.

Torn ligament

A ligament is the tough tissue within a joint that connects muscle to bone or cartilage. If a joint — most likely the knee — is twisted or wrenched, the ligament may be torn. If this occurs, the knee will be tender to the touch and will also hurt when the leg is moved out and to the side. RICE is the first order of business. The injury should also be wrapped for support, with the bandage stretching at least six inches beyond the joint in both directions. Then seek medical care. If this injury does not heal correctly, the knee may remain unstable. Like torn cartilage, this injury is associated with soccer, skiing, and track and field.

Turf toe

Turf toe, also called black nail, is marked by a painful, black toenail. This minor injury occurs when the toes are jammed into the ground, perhaps because the foot is sliding ahead in an ill-fitting shoe and hitting the front of it. This jamming of the toe bruises it and causes blood to collect under the nail. As the name implies, it happens often to athletes playing on artificial turf. First aid is RICE and anti-inflammatory drugs, such as ibuprofen. Pressure under the nail can be released by drilling a heated sterile needle through the nail, which releases a spurt of blood. While this sounds a little gory, the process is quite painless. Be careful, however, to keep the wound clean after the procedure to prevent infection.

Part V
Special Cases

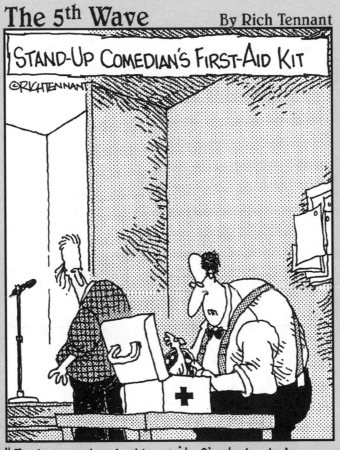

The 5th Wave   By Rich Tennant

STAND-UP COMEDIAN'S FIRST-AID KIT

"Let me check the kit first just in case you bomb. 2 rubber chickens...1 kazoo.. a pair of funny shoes...some nitrous oxide...the musical lyrics to 'Laugh, Clown, Laugh'...3 whoopee cushions..."

In this part . . .

First-aid techniques are not like tube socks: One size does not fit all. With kids, for example, first aid must be tailored to their smaller size. Seniors often have more fragile bones or a greater risk of infection, concerns that must be taken into account. If a person has a disability, that must be considered when providing first aid. Even people in certain occupations have particular risks and needs that go along with their positions. While no single source can cover all of the sizes and shapes of first aid, this part provides an overview of some of the special concerns of the elderly, children, people with disabilities, pregnant women, and office workers and fills you in on how to help them best.

Chapter 23

Special Needs of the Elderly

*G*rowing older means growing wiser, but it also means paying more attention to your health. As birthdays come and go, the body begins to change in some subtle and not-so-subtle ways. These changes may make a person more susceptible to an injury or accident requiring first aid, or they may make a difference in how a person is treated in an emergency situation. In this chapter, you'll find out about what those changes are and how they can affect health. In the following chapter, the discussion continues with a look at specific conditions that may creep up on you with the years.

Changes That Come with Age

While everyone is different, here are some changes that might affect some older people and make them more prone to accidents and conditions requiring first aid.

Decreased sensitivity

As a person gets older, the sense of touch becomes a little less sensitive as nerves become deadened by years of wear and tear. This means Grandma might burn herself taking the cookies out of the oven and not even notice it until later. Or perhaps a senior might be scalded with too-hot tap water, not feeling it until it's too late.

Declines in vision and hearing

Not every senior automatically suffers poor vision or a loss of hearing, but these conditions are common in the elderly. Older adults are more likely to have eye conditions such as cataracts, glaucoma, and retinal diseases, while one-third of Americans between ages 65 and 74 and one-half of those age 85 and older have hearing problems, according to the National Institute on Aging (NIA).

A decline in vision may mean more trips and falls and other injuries, as navigating the home becomes more difficult. Driving may become tougher, too. Even taking medications gets risky if you can't read the label or directions accurately.

With hearing loss, a person might not hear the doctor's directions or may become socially withdrawn or embarrassed about the condition.

Increased inactivity

There's no reason a healthy senior should slow down, but yet the NIA reports that only about one in four older adults exercises regularly, possibly because many older people think they are too old or too frail to exercise.

Unfortunately, the body needs to work out regularly. Without exercise, muscle tone and coordination suffer, the heart rate decreases, circulation slows, and arteries become stiffened and susceptible to blockage. What's more, it keeps confidence and self-esteem up. Without it, a person leaves herself or himself open to heart disease, high blood pressure, arthritis, osteoporosis, increased risk of falls, and a host of other ills.

Decline in cognitive abilities

Cognitive abilities simply means the ability to think clearly. It seems everyone suffers a minor memory lapse now and then as they grow older, but in a small percentage, the problem progresses beyond that. Because of diseases — such as Parkinson's or Alzheimer's — or other conditions or factors, some older adults may lose their short- or long-term memories or even become confused about where they are and what they're doing. Risks associated with this condition include suffering more frequent falls or even malnutrition (if a person fails to eat) or taking improper medications or taking medications improperly.

Decreased circulation

As a person gets older, circulation — the rate at which blood flows throughout the body — slows down. This results in slower healing, increased risk of infection, and changes in the way the body regulates temperature. It may be more difficult for a person to stay warm or cool off in hot weather.

More medical complaints

Heart disease. Diabetes. Cancer. Arthritis. While old age doesn't mean you'll have one of these conditions, it does mean you're more likely to have to face them. That means you'll be more likely to need first aid, too — and not just because you're battling a condition. More conditions mean more drugs, which means a greater chance of a medication error or side effects.

Loss of mobility

Let's face it: While some 70-year-olds out there can run a marathon or do a double back-flip, most people become less agile with age. This might happen because of a lack of exercise or the onset of arthritis, osteoporosis, or another medical condition. Medications taken for various conditions may also cause dizziness or disorientation that makes people less light on their feet. The result is a greater risk of trips, falls, and other injuries.

Weakening of the immune system

The immune system is another function that tends to decline with age, making it harder for the body to fight off the bugs that might invade it. A weakened immune system means that illnesses may be more severe, that they'll last longer, or that they'll more often lead to complications. A bout of the flu, for example, may lead to pneumonia. Or a brush with food poisoning (which healthy adults can fight off within a few days) may cause damage to the kidneys and even death.

Safety in the Home

Just as a home might need to be made safe for a child, some changes might also be in order if there's a senior in your household. Granted, an older adult isn't going to be leaving toys scattered on the floor, but decreases in vision, hearing, and mobility mean you might want to take a few precautions to make things easier to navigate safely:

- **Light up:** Make sure halls and stairways are well-lit and that the lights can be turned on and off from either end. Install lights at all entrances for when you're coming and going. Night lights, flashlights, and luminous tape can make nighttime trips to the bathroom easier, too.

- **Watch your step:** Because falls are common in older adults, take steps to eliminate them. Stairs should have handrails — and you may even want them in your shower or tub. Keep floors uncluttered and electrical cords out of the way. Rugs should be slip-proof — low-pile is a better choice than plush for safety.

- **Keep kitchens cool:** To prevent burns, make sure the stove has lights to show when burners are turned on, and adjust the water heater to prevent tap water from reaching scalding temperatures. Pot handles should be kept turned away from the edge of the stove, and potholders should be kept on hand.

- **Regulate temperatures:** On hot days, make sure air conditioning and fans are being used, and on cold days, check to see if heating is adequate. Older people often don't sense temperatures accurately and may find themselves suddenly overheated or underheated, and all too often they think they can live without air conditioning and hope, instead, to save money. Unfortunately, this can have deadly consequences.

- **Plan for emergencies:** Mark emergency phone numbers in large, readable print near the telephone so seniors can read them clearly. Also make sure your emergency evacuation plans (in the event of a fire, for example), take the needs of an elderly person in mind. Are there any stairs to navigate? Is there an easier route that could be planned?

- **Get connected:** For an older person living alone, you might want to consider a monitoring service that helps keep an eye on things. Some companies offer a button or alarm that can be activated in the case of an emergency — especially one where the person can't get to the phone. Yes, everyone does kid about that catch-phrase "Help, I've fallen, and I can't get up," but the situation is really no laughing matter. To find such a service, contact the local Area Agency on Aging near you (listed in the blue pages of the phone book). A fee is usually involved.

If a professional service isn't an option in your area, ask about nonprofit groups for seniors that may offer an alternative. Some, for example, may arrange to call the elderly person a few times a day to check in and make sure all is well.

Just when you thought you were safe: A look at crime

About 2 million older adults become victims of crime each year. They're often the targets of theft, burglary, and assault, and they're more likely to be confronted by strangers than younger people. Also, caretakers, relatives, and friends may physically, emotionally, or financially abuse elderly people.

To help prevent becoming a victim, seniors should

✔ Put a peephole in the door and refuse to open it for strangers.

✔ Make sure doors and locks are strong.

✔ Keep a record of valuable property — make a list and take pictures of belongings.

✔ Stay alert at all times.

✔ Have pension and Social Security checks deposited directly into an account. This will save a trip to the bank.

✔ Don't carry large amounts of money or valuables with you.

✔ Watch for fraud. Don't give out credit card numbers to people who call on the phone for contributions, don't give people money, and watch out for deals that are "too good to be true." Chances are they're just that.

Safety on the Road

According to the Centers for Disease Control and Prevention, motor-vehicle–related death rates are higher for people 70 years of age and older than for people in any other group except those younger than 25 years.

Why are older people more likely to die in car crashes? Experts say the decline of vision, hearing, cognitive functions, and physical limitations affect driving ability. And because of their age, older people are more likely to die of injuries than people in younger age groups.

During the past decade, the number of drivers over age 70 has increased by almost 50 percent. Because of the aging population, that number is expected to continue to grow.

Older people already have mastered some of the habits that can protect them from injury: Adults over age 70 are more likely to wear seat belts than people in other age groups and they're less likely to drink and drive than younger people. But of course, that doesn't mean you shouldn't be careful. Here are some tips for drivers — both young and old — that could help reduce the risk of injury in a crash:

✔ **Buy a safe car:** Most cars are evaluated to determine how passengers would fare in a crash. To find out if your car is crashworthy, contact the Insurance Institute for Highway Safety, an organization that evaluates cars using crash test dummies in a special testing center. The Institute's address is 1005 N. Glebe Rd., Suite 800, Arlington, VA 22201; (703) 247-1500. They're also on the Web at www.highwaysafety.org.

✔ **Keep your car in good working order:** That way you'll help avoid having breakdowns and getting stranded.

✔ **Use public transportation and only drive when necessary:** The less you're on the road, the less likely it is you'll be in an accident.

✔ **Drive only in the best conditions:** Stay off the roads when it's raining or snowing, or even at night. If you're going to travel to an unfamiliar place at night, take a dry run during the daytime to make sure you know the route.

✔ **Talk with a physician about limitations:** Regular check-ups and tests of vision and hearing can help determine if it's safe for you to be behind the wheel. While it might be hard to give up your independence if your doctor finds you should stop driving, you'll be risking your life (and those of others) if you don't.

Medication Safety

People over age 65 make up 12 percent of the American population, but they take 25 percent of all prescription drugs sold in this country, reports the National Institute on Aging. Older people have more long-term illnesses (such as heart disease and diabetes) and therefore take medications on a long-term basis. Also, older people are likely to have more than one condition, so they may be taking more than one medication for a long period of time.

Drugs — even over-the-counter drugs — are powerful, and they can be harmful if not used correctly. To prevent problems:

✔ Make sure you know how your doctor intends you to use drug — and follow those instructions! Write them down and include them as part of your medical record.

✔ Tell your doctor about all the medications you're taking. (Better yet, pile them in a paper bag and take them to your next doctor visit so that you and she can inventory them together.) This strategy will go far in helping prevent interactions—if your doctor knows every drug you're on.

✔ Don't adjust dosage or stop taking drugs without consulting with your doctor.

✔ Report any side effects or problems that occur when taking drugs.

✔ Keep medications in properly labeled bottles. Double-check that you're taking the right meds before you take them, and don't take them in the dark, where you can't see what you're doing.

✔ Don't take other people's medications. Everyone reacts to drugs differently, so you might not have the same results.

✔ Don't mix alcohol with your medication — it may result in unwanted side effects.

More Information, Please

A host of services are available to older adults. Some provide meals to those who no longer cook. Some provide medical equipment for those who need help getting around. Still others help with health and insurance issues, providing valuable information and resources to older adults and their families.

A good place to start is your local Area Agency on Aging, a government organization dedicated to providing services for older adults. To find the agency near you, use their Eldercare Locator at (800) 677-1116.

Another option is the National Institute for Aging, part of the National Institutes of Health. It operates a toll-free information line at (800) 222-2225. You can also find information on health and aging on their Web site at www.nih.gov/nia.

Need more options? Here are some other resources you may find helpful:

✔ American Association of Homes and Services for the Aging, 901 E. St., N.W., Suite 500, Washington, DC 20004; (202) 783-2242, www.aahsa.org

✔ National Association of Meals Program, 101 N. Alfred St., Suite 202, Alexandria, VA 22314; (703) 548-5558

✔ National Council on Aging, 409 Third St., S.W., Washington, DC 20024; (202) 479-1200, www.ncoa.org

Chapter 24

Unique Problems of the Elderly

- -

- -

*I*t might be a burn. It might be a nasty fall. Whatever the case, you find yourself face to face with an elderly victim in need of first aid. What do you do? For the most part, you use the tried-and-true first-aid procedures you rely on in every emergency situation. But seniors do have some special needs you'll want to address — and that's what this chapter is all about.

On the Scene: Do's and Don'ts

When faced with providing first aid to an older person, here are some do's and don'ts to keep in mind.

- ✔ **Don't talk down to the victim:** Some people see — and treat — seniors as if they were children, but that's hardly the case. Older people have a great deal of knowledge and expertise and shouldn't be written off.

- ✔ **Don't assume the victim is hard of hearing:** A decline in hearing is far from automatic in older adults, so don't begin first aid by shouting at the victim. It won't be appreciated.

- ✔ **Do communicate clearly:** In any emergency situation, it's important to explain to the victim exactly what you're doing at all times.

- ✔ **Don't be rough:** With age often comes brittle bones and fragile skin, so take care to be gentle when providing first aid for older victims. Too much pressure could result in bruises or even broken bones.

- ✔ **Do be patient:** An older person may take longer to respond to your questions and comments than you expect, but don't rush. Give the person a chance to communicate thoughts and feelings in his or her own time.

- ✔ **Do remain calm:** Some older people are set in their ways, so an injury or accident can be especially upsetting.

What to Watch For

As was said in Chapter 23, seniors tend to become more susceptible to certain conditions as they age. In fact, a number of health problems requiring first aid are common in older adults. What are they? Glad you asked . . .

Allergies

Experts have found that elderly people tend to have more severe reactions to insect venom, which makes bee stings and other bites a risk for them. Signs of severe reaction include

- ✔ Itching
- ✔ Hives
- ✔ Dizziness
- ✔ Nausea
- ✔ Difficulty breathing
- ✔ Difficulty swallowing
- ✔ Unconsciousness

If the person has allergy medicine, help him or her take it. An Epi-Pen — an already prepared syringe of epinephrine, available by prescription only — is one "antidote" to allergic reactions. Follow the instructions on the pen to administer the medication. You can find more on bites and stings in Chapter 13.

Bruises

Blood vessels become fragile with age. In some seniors, even a firm grasp of an arm or leg or a light bump against the sofa might yield a bruise. Treat minor bruises with an ice pack wrapped in a towel to prevent swelling and ask a physician to check more severe bumps to ensure there's no internal bleeding.

Burns

Burns are common in older people because they tend to be less sensitive to heat. As a result, a senior might grasp a hot pot handle or brush up against a hot radiator, not noticing until damage has been done. First aid for burns in seniors is no different than treatment for others, although it may take them longer to heal.

Choking

Choking is common in seniors for a few reasons. First, just as the hands and skin may become less sensitive, so might the mouth and tongue, which increases the risk of choking. Dentures also make a person more prone to choking — although the alternative of eating without dentures is also dangerous. Food may not be chewed enough or reduced enough in size to be readily swallowed.

If choking occurs, the Heimlich maneuver is the most appropriate move. Try to be gentle, but make sure you provide enough force to be effective. Of course, between a fractured rib and a death by choking, the rib is the lesser of the two evils.

Difficulty breathing

Difficulty breathing is really a symptom rather than a condition. In the elderly, it may be one of the first signs of serious illness. If a senior is having trouble breathing and there's no apparent condition, seek medical attention. Keep a close eye on vital signs (heart and breathing rates) and be prepared to begin cardiopulmonary resuscitation (CPR) if the need arises.

Fractures

According to the Centers for Disease Control and Prevention, of all deaths associated with falls, 60 percent involve people age 75 years or older. For people age 65 years or older, 60 percent of fatal falls occur in the home, 30 percent occur in public places, and 10 percent occur in health care institutions.

It may seem strange that something as simple as a fall can cause death. But the problem usually isn't the fall itself. It's the inability of the body to recover from the broken bone. A hip injury, for example, might not heal properly and the victim may remain in bed for months, gradually becoming weaker, until an infection or other condition takes advantage.

Factors that contribute to falls in older people include a decline in vision, nerve and muscle problems, disorienting medications, and difficulties in gait and balance. Environmental hazards such as slippery surfaces, uneven floors, poor lighting, loose rugs, unstable furniture, and objects on floors may also play a role.

If a fall occurs and causes injury, follow the guidelines in Chapter 20 on handling a bone or joint problem. If the person must be transported, see Chapter 7 for emergency transfer information.

Osteoporosis

Osteoporosis is a condition that causes bones to weaken, making them likely to break even under little pressure. It usually occurs in older people — especially women — when the body lacks the vitamins and minerals it needs to build strong bones.

The condition is fairly common: One out of two women and one in eight men over age 50 will have an osteoporosis-related fracture, says the National Institute on Aging. Prevention means getting enough calcium, exercising regularly (strength exercises are especially helpful), and getting enough vitamin D, especially when you're younger.

Osteoporosis is one reason you need to be gentle when performing first aid on an older person. Chest compressions, the Heimlich maneuver, or even just moving someone roughly can cause a fractured bone.

Heat-related illness

Of the people who die each year from heat-related illnesses, most are over 50 years of age, says the National Institute on Aging. But why are seniors so susceptible to conditions such as heat stroke and heat exhaustion? For one thing, they're more likely to suffer from poor circulation, inefficient sweat glands, lung and heart diseases, and high blood pressure, all of which increase the risk of heat-related illness. For another, some types of medications, such as salt pills, diuretics, and blood pressure drugs, also increase risk.

Seniors also tend to be reluctant to really make use of air conditioning, perhaps because they're so used to living without it, or because they're afraid of how the electric bill might balloon. Don't be hesitant, though, to turn the A/C on and turn it up. Whatever it costs, it's worth it for your health.

With heat-related illness, seniors tend to go from feeling fine to sudden collapse, so when dealing with an older person with a heat-related illness, don't hesitate to seek medical attention.

Hypothermia

Older people tend to have less effective circulation and to be in poorer heath, which increases chances of hypothermia — lowered body temperature. Or they make take medications that interfere with body's ability to regulate temperature.

TIP

Getting warmed up

Hypothermia isn't something that only happens on the frozen tundra. It could happen in your own home. That's right! Just sitting still in a too-cool room might lower a senior's body temperature enough that hypothermia sets in.

To prevent hypothermia:

✔ Keep the home warm, more than 65 degrees F. Make sure insulation and weatherproofing is adequate. Your power company may have a program to help you winterize your home. If heating bills are a concern, check with your local government. Many locations provide financial support for those who need help paying heating costs.

✔ Keep an eye on health. Some illnesses place a person at risk because they affect the way the body handles cold temperatures. Conditions that may blunt the response to

cold include hypothyroidism and other disorders of the body's hormone system, stroke, severe arthritis, Parkinson's disease, memory disorders, or other illnesses that limit activity or slow circulation.

✔ Watch your medications. Certain medicines increase the risk of accidental hypothermia. They include drugs used to treat anxiety, depression, or nausea, and some over-the-counter cold remedies. Ask your doctor how your medicines affect body heat.

✔ Stay away from caffeine and alcohol. In addition to some medications, alcoholic and caffeinated drinks lower the body's ability to retain heat. Hot chocolate or coffee may make you *feel* warmer temporarily, but your true body temperature may actually decrease.

Infection

Older people tend to be more susceptible to infections as their immune systems gradually slow down. As a result, conditions that a younger person might shrug off in a matter of days — such as the flu or food poisoning — can cause serious complications for seniors.

First aid for infection generally means seeking medical care as soon as possible once symptoms of illness or infection appear. The sooner a doctor evaluates the situation, the better the outcome tends to be.

Of course, an ounce of prevention is worth a pound of cure, and there's plenty of prevention to go around in this category. Seniors should make sure to get a pneumonia vaccine, for one thing. That one little shot should protect against 88 percent of all pneumococcal bacteria for up to ten years. Another must is the flu shot, which should be administered annually by mid-November. Tetanus and diphtheria vaccinations are also important, and other shots might be recommended for people in certain circumstances. For example, a health care worker may be smart to get a hepatitis B vaccination.

Poisoning

Older people have more medications to take and often must deal with poor eyesight and small labels. That means there's more of a chance that medications will be mixed up or taken in the wrong dosages — or even not taken at all, if a person becomes forgetful. The other risk is that an older person will accidentally ingest a harmful substance, again perhaps because of poor eyesight or mental confusion.

Signs of poisoning are

- Rash on the skin or around the mouth
- Headache
- Chills or fever
- Numbness
- Painful swallowing
- Nausea and abdominal problems
- Contracted pupils (this means they're very tight and small)
- Blurred vision
- Difficulty breathing
- Chest pain and heart palpitations

If you suspect poisoning, contact your poison control center as soon as possible for first aid instructions. See Chapter 12 for more on poisoning.

Stroke

According to the National Institute on Aging, the death rate from stroke is down about 50 percent in the past decade. However, it is still the third leading cause of death in the United States and the leading cause of disability in adults.

The elderly are at a greater risk of stroke because they tend to have high blood pressure and heart disease. A person interested in preventing stroke should stop smoking, control blood pressure, exercise regularly, eat well, and control diabetes, if appropriate.

The key to first aid and stroke is to get medical attention to the victim as soon as possible. The sooner treatment begins, the less the damage to the brain. For more details, see Chapter 19.

Chapter 25

Special Needs of Children

● ●

● ●

Almost every parent ends up in the emergency room with a crying child on the lap at least once while his or her kid is growing up. In fact, statistics show that kids are notoriously accident prone. The Centers for Disease Control and Prevention say that every 2½ minutes in the United States, roughly one preschool or elementary school student visits the ER after an injury on playground equipment. Further, they report that each year 20 to 25 percent of all children sustain an injury serious enough to need medical attention. And while unintentional injuries — caused by fires, car accidents, drownings, falls, poisonings, and the like — rarely cause death, they're still the leading cause of fatal accidents in kids. This chapter looks at the reasons behind injuries in children, and how you can help head them off before they strike.

What's the Problem with Kids These Days?

Looking at our television stereotypes, like Dennis the Menace, Bart Simpson, and (of course) Wally and the Beaver, it's not hard to imagine why kids are likely to end up in the doctor's office or emergency room. Yet it's not just destiny that kids are accident prone — they have certain characteristics and limitations that need to be taken into consideration when it comes to safety.

✔ **Kids are pretty active:** As an adult, you may find yourself in a temperature-controlled office facing a desk or computer screen. But as a kid, you're out and about on the playground and in the neighborhood, riding a bike or roughhousing with your friends. And that's a lifestyle that leaves you prone to skinned knees, broken bones, and a host of other injuries.

- ✔ **Kids aren't that smart (yet):** Not to insult their intelligence, but the truth is that there's a lot about the way the world works that kids just don't know or understand — for example, why it's not a good idea to put a fork in the electrical socket or sit on a younger sibling's head. Don't trust them to follow their common sense — that's something that must come with age and experience.

- ✔ **Kids are smarter than you think:** Yes, this contradicts the previous point, but children are funny creatures. Even though they can't tie their own shoes, they may manage to understand the mechanics of the cap to the laundry detergent or the button to the garage door opener — another reason to keep an eye out for safety.

- ✔ **Kids explore:** Curiosity killed the cat, but it could also cause a risk to your child. One reason kids seem to be into everything all the time is that they're exploring — new sights, new sounds, new tastes, and new sensations. Should these Columbus-esque behaviors cross paths with, say, a hazardous substance, you've got yourself a problem.

- ✔ **Kids aren't mature yet:** It's an obvious point, but one that bears repeating in this context. Small bones are more fragile, small bodies are more susceptible to poisons, and small immune systems are more likely to succumb to germs and other hazards. In addition, different stages of growth bring awkwardness as kids get used to their physical abilities. And when they do master the way their bodies work, they often overestimate what they can do with them. For this reason, experts say, accident rates peak around third grade.

What's the solution to these childlike tendencies? Childproofing your home and any play areas is one healthy solution (which will be discussed in a second). But your best bet is to give your kids the attention they need. In other words, keep an eye on them until they're able to keep an eye out for themselves.

Proofing for Prevention

Childproofing your house is an obvious way to keep accidents to a minimum. While a book on first aid isn't really the place to go into great detail about all you can do to create a safe environment for your kids — and there's plenty you could do — here are some quick tips to get you started.

Protecting baby

Infants are rarely out of a parent's sight and thankfully don't have the run of the house. Still, you should take a few precautions to ensure your infant's safety.

✔ Make sure the crib is safe. A crib should have no sharp edges and a locking mechanism to keep the sides in place. The distance from the top of the rail to the mattress should be at least 26 inches when the mattress is at its lowest level. The mattress should fit snugly, and bumper pads should be in place. A pillow is not necessary. If you're using an antique or second-hand crib, make sure it's up to safety requirements. Also, fluffy pillows and blankets can cause suffocation, so it's best not to use them in a crib.

✔ Keep plastic bags away from your baby. Young children can suffocate while playing with plastic bags.

✔ Select only fireproof blankets and pajamas.

✔ Make sure any mobiles above the crib are secure and out of the infant's reach.

✔ Toys should be large and soft. Avoid toys with buttons or parts that can be swallowed. Follow age recommendations on products.

✔ Watch out for subtle risks. For example, the cords that hang down from draperies pose a choking risk, so check their length.

Taming toddlers

Once kids get to their feet, childproofing becomes a lot more challenging. In this stage of life:

✔ Restrict access for your child. Use baby gates and lock or guard accessible windows. Then concentrate on childproofing the rooms your child has access to.

✔ Cover electrical outlets with safety caps, available at hardware and children's stores.

✔ Store hazardous substances out of reach. These include cleaning products, insecticides, medications, and matches. Install childproof locks on cabinets. Watch out for plants, too — these can be poisonous if swallowed, although most people don't think of them as a hazard.

✔ Practice burn safety. In the kitchen, keep pot handles pointed toward the stove, don't leave hot beverages near the edge of a table (or drink one while carrying your child), and adjust your water heater to prevent tap water from scalding little hands.

✔ Watch out for water. Keep the lid down on the toilet seat. Believe it or not, even that small amount of water presents a drowning danger. And, of course, don't leave your toddler alone in the bathtub or baby pool.

These tips are only the tip of the iceberg, so to speak, when it comes to child-proofing. More on safety can be found in Chapters 1 and 2, but for a complete discussion, check out some of the many books on the subject at your local library or bookstore, or ask your pediatrician for advice.

Surviving the great outdoors

Once you've give your house a once-over, check out the yard. Here are some suggestions to keep in mind:

- Have your child play where you can monitor activities.
- Use grass, wood chips, sand, or other soft surfaces under swing sets and play equipment to soften any falls.
- Make sure equipment is properly assembled and anchored to prevent tipping.
- Keep any toys and equipment in good condition. Rough wood can cause slivers, and rusty spots can lead to tetanus.
- Establish ground rules. For example, one person on the swing at a time, hold on with both hands, no standing or kneeling allowed.

Passing on Your Knowledge

As kids get older, be sure to share with them the do's and don'ts of your household, and the reasons behind them. As was said before, common sense comes with age and experience, and pointing out dangers helps give your child a firm foundation for future safety.

But kids don't just need to know about prevention — they need to know how to take action if an emergency strikes.

Most important, kids (even young ones) need to know how to call for help. Have your child memorize emergency numbers and keep those numbers (along with your address) next to the phone. Also let kids know that, in a pinch, they can always simply dial "0" for help. Teach them — as early as they're able to accomplish this — their own address and phone number.

Have your child practice calling for help with an unplugged phone, just to see that he or she has the hang of it. Explain an imaginary scenario (Mom fell down and hit her head) and have the child go through the motions of calling while you play the part of the operator, asking questions that EMS might ask. The exercise will show your child what to expect if a call needs to be made and ease any fears about calling for help.

Also make sure your kids know what to do in case of fire. Kids should be taught a few basics: shout if you see or smell a fire; get out of the house right away — don't stop to save toys or try to hide in a closet; and stop, drop, and roll if clothes should happen to ignite. As a family, decide on a meeting place if a fire occurs (for example, by the stop sign on the corner or some such place). And test out your fire alarms so kids know what they sound like.

Whatever you do, don't underestimate the talents of kids in an emergency. If you're attending a victim, remember that a child can sometimes be sent for help if you can't get away. Often, too, they can follow instructions from EMS to provide lifesaving first aid.

Chapter 26

Unique Problems of Children

• •

• •

*W*ith kids always on the go, don't be surprised if an accident involving one stops you in your tracks. But taking care of a child in an emergency can be trying — after all, you're dealing with a victim who might not be able to understand what's going on, follow your instructions, or maybe even express himself or herself clearly. Plus, you'll need to alter some of your first-aid techniques to accommodate your pint-sized "patient." Fortunately, that's what this chapter is all about.

On the Scene: Do's and Don'ts

Approaching a victim who's a child is different than dealing with an adult or an elderly person, and you need to adjust your actions and demeanor accordingly. Here are some do's and don'ts that could make providing first aid easier and safer:

✔ **Do seek consent:** You may remember seeing this in Chapter 3. The rule with kids under age 18 is that you need to ask a parent or guardian for consent *before* you begin first aid. If the guardian doesn't want you to provide aid, you must abide by those wishes. However, if no one is around to give that consent, you may assume *implied consent* — that the guardian would give permission if present.

✔ **Don't act nervous or scared:** It's cliché, but true. Kids can sense fear, and if you're frightened, the child is going to be scared, too. Do your best to squash your fears when providing first aid to a young patient, and act calm and confident. The more relaxed you are, the more relaxed the child will be, and his or her breathing or heart rate will be slower. Be upbeat, too, to avoid tears. It's better to say "You'll be okay!" than draw attention to the injury with an "Oh, that must hurt!"

✔ **Do talk on the child's level — literally:** Hunker down next to any little victims so you can see them and talk to them on their own level. Towering above your patient will only increase stress.

✔ **Do make contact:** Look the child in the eye and maybe give the kid a pat on the head or a touch on the shoulder for reassurance.

✔ **Don't get frustrated:** Kids can't always tell you what happened, and they may not even be able to tell you "where it hurts." Do the best with the information you have, and leave the rest to medical professionals where appropriate.

✔ **Do explain your actions:** Whether you're wrapping a bandage or calling for help, take the time to tell the child what you're doing and how you're doing it. For example, you might show the child the scissors, bandages, and antiseptic you're going to use to clean up a small wound. The courtesy will make the child more comfortable.

✔ **Don't underestimate kids:** While treating a child with first aid may be different than treating an adult, you should treat them both the same when it comes to respect. While you should keep your explanations simple, try not to talk down to the child or underestimate the amount of pain he or she is in. Just do your best to comfort and reassure.

Tailoring Techniques

Because of the differences between infants, children, and adults, first-aid techniques need to be adapted to take into account kids' smaller statures and more vulnerable bodies.

One difference is in taking the pulse. With an adult, you'd probably go for the pulse point in the wrist or at the side of the neck. With a child under 1 year old, however, the recommended pulse point is on the inside of the upper arm — a point called the *brachial* pulse point. To take a pulse in an infant, gently press two fingers on the inside of the arm, between the elbow and the shoulder, and feel for 5 to 10 seconds.

Another difference is the way CPR is provided. Depending on the age of the child, the number of breaths and chest compressions varies, so make sure you take age into consideration. Chapter 19 covers the details on these variations.

You also have to handle first aid for choking differently. Obviously, you can't apply the rough Heimlich maneuver to an infant. So the solution is a method involving back blows and chest compressions administered with only two fingers. Chapter 15 offers illustrations and instructions on this method.

Finally, take into consideration a child's age when dealing with medications. Even over-the-counter drugs are powerful, and in the wrong dosage, they can be harmful to young bodies. Be sure to carefully follow package instructions or the instructions of your child's health care provider.

This is just an overview of some of the differences in first-aid techniques. For specifics on all injuries and how to handle them, consult the appropriate chapters in this book.

Knowing What to Watch For

The way they're built, along with their habits and activities, puts kids at higher risk for some types of injuries and conditions. Here's a quick rundown of some of the most common problems children might encounter.

Allergies

Like elderly people, infants and children tend to have more severe reactions to insect venom than healthy adults, which makes bee stings and other bites a risk for them. Kids are also more likely to get stung because they're often outdoors, somewhat low to the ground, and less likely to leave "sleeping bees lie." Signs of severe reaction include

- ✔ Itching
- ✔ Hives
- ✔ Dizziness
- ✔ Nausea
- ✔ Difficulty breathing
- ✔ Difficulty swallowing
- ✔ Unconsciousness

If the child has allergy medicine, help him or her take it. An Epi-Pen — an already prepared syringe of epinephrine, available by prescription only — is one "antidote" to allergic reactions. Follow the instructions on the pen to administer the medication. More on bites and stings can be found in Chapter 13.

Bone and joint injuries

You've all seen the public service ads pushing calcium and milk for children. Kids need calcium because they're continually growing. Their bones and muscles need the proper nutrients if they're going to become as strong as they can be. But the point here is that, during formative years, bones are somewhat brittle and muscles are easily stretched and pulled — even rough-housing in the backyard may lead to accidental injury.

If injured, check out Chapter 20, and be sure to seek medical attention. One up-side to childhood is that kids heal quickly, but injuries need to be attended to the right way if they're going to heal properly.

Poisoning

A combination of curiosity and ignorance contributes to the fact that kids under the age of 6 account for 53 percent of all cases of poisoning. Unfortunately, because of their small body size, kids are more susceptible to the effects of poisoning as toxins spread quickly through the bloodstream. If you suspect poisoning, call the poison control center hot line as soon as possible, and be sure to tell the operator that the victim is a child. Report age and approximate weight so you can get precise instructions on how to provide first aid. Chapter 12 covers details on poisoning.

When talking about poisoning, don't forget about food poisoning. Children don't have the fully developed immune systems that will come with age, so unfriendly bugs in the system — which can come from eating undercooked or contaminated foods — may quickly take over. The possibilities are a little frightening. An exposure to foodborne bacteria that may only cause stomach cramps in an adult may cause serious injury or even death in a child. Seek medical care immediately if you suspect food poisoning.

To help prevent, follow food safety guidelines. Cook all meats and poultry thoroughly (don't leave the burgers medium-rare), store foods at a proper temperature, wash fruits and vegetables before serving, and store any left-overs promptly after the meal is over.

Infection

The not-yet-developed immune system — the same loophole in kids that lets food poisoning creep in — also leaves children open to other germs that cause infection. To help prevent infections, turn to the old standbys such as washing hands, covering open wounds with bandages, and avoiding exposure to contaminated pals. If infection strikes — and it surely will — get advice from your child's health care practitioner on how to handle it.

Vomiting and diarrhea

Often, the risk with vomiting and diarrhea is not the bug that's causing it, but with the dehydration that it's causing your child. Kids are very sensitive to dehydration and lose water rapidly if they're throwing up or having repeated bouts of diarrhea. As with food poisoning, these symptoms might just mean discomfort in adults, but can be life-threatening in children. Seek care right away if it persists for any length of time.

Heat illness and hypothermia

Here are two other conditions that may cause children risk, thanks to their underdeveloped body systems. In this case, temperature regulation is the culprit. Young children's sweat glands aren't yet developed (not until puberty), so they can't cool off as easily as adults. On the other hand, their heat-conserving mechanisms aren't in full force yet either, so they lose heat easily through their skin. This means that in both hot and cold temps, you need to keep a close eye on your child. On summer days, don't hesitate to call for a time-out in the shade. In the winter, force hats and mittens on the youngsters. At the same time, watch for symptoms of temperature-related illness. See Chapter 16 for details on exposure to cold and Chapter 17 for details on heat-related illness.

Chapter 27

First Aid During Pregnancy and Childbirth

*P*regnancy is a challenge, both physically and emotionally. Not only is a woman's body undergoing impressive changes during the nine months before she gives birth, she's also going through a wide range of emotions — from amazement to anxiety.

While this chapter can't ease worries about the financial or career obstacles pregnancy presents, it can help reduce apprehension about how to handle some of the problems that may arise during pregnancy and childbirth. You'll also find information on what to do If you're faced with an emergency delivery (so you won't have to rely on your vague recollections of *Gone With the Wind*).

Ectopic Pregnancy

Ectopic pregnancy is a rare, life-threatening condition that strikes very early in pregnancy. Also called tubal pregnancy, it occurs when the fertilized egg begins to grow somewhere outside the *uterus* (or womb), where it belongs. Most often, a misplaced egg implants on a fallopian tube, but it may also settle on an ovary or in the abdominal cavity. The problem occurs when the egg begins to develop, rupturing the fallopian tube or other tissues and causing internal bleeding. The condition cannot be prevented.

Ectopic pregnancy is a serious condition; without immediate medical attention, it may cause death. According to the Centers for Disease Control and Prevention, the condition is rare, comprising 2 percent of all pregnancies.

The factors that make ectopic pregnancy more likely for a woman include

- An age of 30 years or more
- Previous abdominal or fallopian tube surgery
- Smoking
- Use of the fertility procedure called gamete intrafallopian transfer (GIFT)

Also, if ectopic pregnancy has occurred in the past, it's more likely to occur again.

Symptoms

The condition occurs during the first few weeks after conception, and many women who have it may not even know they're pregnant. Symptoms include

- Cramps
- Vaginal bleeding
- Severe lower abdominal pains on one side of the body
- Nausea and vomiting
- Fainting spells
- Dizziness

Soothing morning sickness

Granted, morning sickness is not an emergency that requires first aid, but knowing how to handle it can make pregnancy much easier on a woman.

Morning sickness, by definition, is nausea and vomiting that occurs in the first three months after conception. It doesn't always happen in the morning but also in the evening. It may come on stronger at mealtimes. If weight loss occurs because of morning sickness, seek medical attention. Hospitalization and intravenous feeding may be necessary in severe cases.

To help curb nausea and vomiting, a woman should eat small, frequent meals. Drinking plenty of water and juice can help prevent dehydration and also soothe symptoms. One natural remedy is ginger tea, thought to ease nausea.

First to last

First aid for ectopic pregnancy is the same as for any closed wound: Call for medical help immediately. Don't move the affected part of the body. Also, don't give the woman any food or water — even if she complains of being thirsty.

The condition is hard to diagnose and may require an ultrasound (a procedure that uses sound waves to create an image of the internal tissues) or laparoscopy (a procedure in which a thin scope is inserted into the abdomen to take a look around). Medical treatment includes surgery to remove the misplaced egg and repair damaged tissues. Ectopic pregnancy always results in the loss of the pregnancy.

Miscarriage

Miscarriage is the loss of a pregnancy before the fetus is sufficiently developed. It occurs in 15 to 20 percent of all pregnancies and is most likely in women over the age of 35. Most miscarriages occur before the 12th week of pregnancy and are caused by an abnormality in the way the fetus is developing or in the woman's body.

A number of factors put a woman at risk for miscarriage. They include

- ✔ A weakened cervix (the opening of the uterus)
- ✔ An age of 35 years or older
- ✔ An illness such as diabetes or high blood pressure
- ✔ Obesity
- ✔ A hormonal or genetic disorder
- ✔ An anatomical abnormality in the uterus

Like ectopic pregnancy, miscarriage is more likely to occur if it has happened in the past.

Miscarriage is *not* caused by activities such as jumping, exercising, or having sex. It's not brought on by stress and emotional shock, and very rarely does it occur because of trauma.

Symptoms

A small amount of bleeding may occur in the very early stages of pregnancy — within the first ten days after fertilization has occurred. This is normal, and no cause for alarm. However, if the bleeding persists longer than two days, seek medical attention. Typical signs of miscarriage include

- Vaginal bleeding
- Severe abdominal pain
- Severe cramps
- Fever
- Pressure or pain in the lower back
- Abdominal or thigh pain that comes and goes
- Unusual vaginal discharge, or discharge that appears to contain tissue

Although pain and cramping usually accompany miscarriage, it may be painless in some women.

First to last

Seek medical care immediately if you suspect miscarriage. In some cases, it may be able to be prevented. If possible, keep any tissue that has been passed. It may be used to help determine the cause of the miscarriage.

When Push Comes to Shove: Labor and Delivery

Nine months of waiting precedes the delivery of a child, but labor and childbirth may start unexpectedly and progress quickly — before there's time to get medical care. That's when first-aid skills come in handy.

Some people say there's not much to having a baby. After all, women have been doing it for thousands and thousands of years without much help. And that's essentially right. Statistics show that 90 percent of women can deliver naturally without medical attention. Still, you should be aware of some things if you're on the scene.

Complicating pregnancy

Complications — medical problems that interfere with the health of the woman or her infant during pregnancy — are not common, but they do occur. Here's a quick rundown of some of the most common complications:

✔ **Cervical incompetence:** The *cervix* is the mouth of the uterus, or womb. Usually, it's closed tightly during pregnancy, holding the fetus safely inside. But if it becomes weakened, the infant may be delivered prematurely or the cervix itself may become damaged. The main sign of cervical incompetence is bleeding during pregnancy. If this symptom occurs, report it to your doctor immediately. Cervical incompetence can be treated with bed rest or surgery, and most women with the condition can carry to term if helped in time.

✔ **Gestational diabetes:** This is a fancy way of saying "diabetes that develops during pregnancy." It develops in some nondiabetic women five to seven months into the pregnancy and usually disappears after delivery. Only in 1 to 3 percent of cases will it interfere with a healthy, normal pregnancy. Symptoms include frequent urination, constant thirst and hunger, weight loss, and blurry vision. Tell your doctor if any such signs appear.

✔ **Gestational hypertension:** This is a fancy way of saying "high blood pressure during pregnancy." It usually occurs in women over age 35 and can signal preeclampsia or eclampsia, a toxic condition that occurs late in pregnancy. This condition, which usually has no symptoms, is often discovered by a doctor during a routine blood-pressure check — a good reason to make sure you get proper prenatal care.

✔ **Preeclampsia and eclampsia (toxemia of pregnancy):** These conditions, which occur after the 20th week of pregnancy, are very serious if not treated promptly. Early symptoms, which set in over 24 hours, include high blood pressure, hand and facial swelling, and protein in the urine. As the condition progresses, a woman may have convulsions and go into a coma.

✔ **Rh disease:** Rh disease occurs when a woman and her infant have different types of an immune system substance called Rh factor. The difference causes the woman's immune system to attack and destroy the fetus' blood cells and can result in the loss of the pregnancy. A woman can receive a blood test before pregnancy to see if Rh disease will occur, and get a vaccine if necessary to prevent it. If Rh disease does occur, treatment is possible using blood transfusions.

Symptoms

First, you'll notice symptoms that the baby will be arriving on the scene soon. These include

- ✔ Contractions less than two minutes apart
- ✔ A feeling from the mother that the baby is on the way
- ✔ An urge to push or an urge to have a bowel movement by the mother
- ✔ The baby's head visible within the vagina (a seemingly obvious one)

First to last

In addition to knowing the symptoms, you also know what to have on hand. Pillows, blankets, clean sheets, a plastic sheet (a shower curtain works, too), and towels (or clean newspapers, in a pinch), sanitary napkins, rubber gloves, and a suction bulb (a tool like a miniature turkey-baster that can be picked up at a drugstore) are among the supplies on the list for emergency delivery. After the baby has arrived, you may need a clean pair of scissors, a clean string to tie the umbilical cord, and a plastic bag or container to save the placenta.

If a baby's on the way and you can't get to a hospital, call EMS right away. Even though most women can deliver without assistance, complications do occur at times, so you want EMS to be on the way. Don't try to delay delivery yourself by crossing the mother's legs or blocking the passage of the baby's head — you'll only risk hurting mom and child.

Before delivery

Using soap and water, wash your hands and put on sterile gloves. Then, find a clean place — such as a bed or table — to create a birthing area. Lay down the plastic sheet, then cover it with the clean sheet or clean newspapers or towels.

Next, get the mother into position. If she wants to lie down, support her head and back with pillows and have her spread her legs open. While lying down is a common birthing position, she may alternatively want to squat or lie on one side with one leg raised.

During labor, have the mother breathe deeply and slowly. When the baby's head will become visible in the vagina, you'll want to help the process along by pushing gently on the area below the vagina during contractions. During each contraction, ask the mother to push.

Some blood is normal during childbirth, but heavy bleeding during labor is a sign that something may be wrong. If it occurs, seek emergency care immediately. But how can you tell what's normal and what's excessive? The American Red Cross offers this guideline: one to two cups is normal — any more warrants emergency care.

If the woman is bleeding before the child is born, it may be a sign of *placenta previa,* in which the placenta — the organ that nourishes the fetus while in the womb — blocks the opening of the uterus so the baby can't be delivered. It may also signal *placenta abruptio,* in which the placenta separates from the wall of the uterus prematurely. Both of these conditions are usually handled by cesarean section, a surgical procedure to remove the child through the uterine wall. Seek emergency attention immediately if complications occur.

During delivery

As the child is delivered, support the head with your hands as it appears (see Figure 27-1). The head will appear first, followed by the shoulders. If the baby seems to get stuck at this point, help it along by pushing gently on the lower abdomen, just above the pubic region, while the mother pushes. Don't pull on the baby — let the delivery progress on its own. Once the shoulders are free, the rest of the body will follow quickly, turning to one side. The baby may be slippery, so you may want to use a towel when supporting him.

Again, excessive bleeding — more than one to two cups of blood — requires immediate emergency care. Other problems that may occur during delivery include an out-of-place umbilical cord, a child in an unusual presentation, or the presence of meconium, a greenish-brown material.

- **Umbilical cord complications:** The umbilical cord is the tube through which the infant receives oxygen and nourishment. If it's out of place during delivery, the strong muscular contractions of the mother's uterus may squeeze the cord, cutting off the child's lifeline.

  If the cord is visible in the birth canal before the baby is, or if they both appear at the same time, have the mother kneel, face down, with her knees to her chest and her buttocks in the air. Have her remain in that position until help arrives or you can get her to an emergency room.

  If the cord is wrapped around the baby's neck, try to slip it off over the head. If that can't be done, tie it off in two places, then cut the cord between the two ties.

  Do not cut the cord without tying it off in this way or the infant will bleed to death.

- **Unusual presentation:** *Presentation* refers to the position the child is in when it travels through the birth canal. Most babies are born face down, head-first, but they may also come with a foot, knee, or buttock first.

  To help the infant along, have someone gently press down on the mother's stomach, just above the line of pubic hair. The pressure will speed delivery. Let delivery occur naturally, but watch to make sure the head delivers within three minutes after the shoulders come through. If it does not, gently lift the infant's body (which will be face down) up toward the ceiling. The infant's mouth and nose should appear. Wipe them off to clear them of any mucus, then allow the delivery to progress. *Don't* try to pull the baby out of the vagina.

✔ **Meconium:** Meconium is a bowel movement of a fetus. It only appears when the fetus is in distress — for example, if it's not getting enough oxygen. What's more, the meconium itself may be inhaled by the infant and cause respiratory problems. If you see this brownish-green stuff, seek emergency care immediately.

✔ **Unbroken amniotic sac:** If the baby is still encased in the fluid-filled sac during delivery, tear it open with your fingers. Otherwise, the child will not be able to breathe.

After delivery

If the baby's not breathing when it's delivered, tap the soles of its feet and rub its back. Hold the baby's feet higher than its head, and keep the baby face down. This will help fluids drain (see Figure 27-1). You can also use the suction bulb again to clear fluid and mucus from the nose and mouth of the child. If the child does not begin to breathe, use infant CPR. Instructions on how to perform infant CPR can be found in Chapter 19.

Once the baby is breathing or crying, wipe off the baby (don't wash off the baby), wrap it in a blanket to keep it warm, and place it on its mother's stomach. Encourage the infant to begin nursing, which will stimulate the delivery of the placenta, the organ that nourishes the baby during the pregnancy. Once the placenta is delivered, put it in a plastic bag to take to the hospital with mother and child. If the placenta isn't passed within about a half an hour, seek immediate medical attention because there's a risk that excessive bleeding may occur. Don't pull on the umbilical cord in an attempt to bring out the placenta.

Once the placenta is delivered, tie off the umbilical cord. Use a thick string or shoelace and securely tie it off at least four inches from the child. There's no need to cut the umbilical cord right away. In fact, it's best to leave that up to emergency personnel because of the risk of infection caused by cutting it. If you must cut the cord, first tie another string around the cord another four inches away from the naval, the cut between the knot with sterilized scissors. Bandage the end of the cord with a clean dressing.

Remember: Do not cut the cord without tying it off in this way or the infant will bleed to death.

After the delivery, massage the mother's abdomen to encourage more contractions, which will expel any blood or fluids from the uterus. If the mother is bleeding from a tear in the opening of the vagina, keep pressure on the area with a sanitary napkin until bleeding stops.

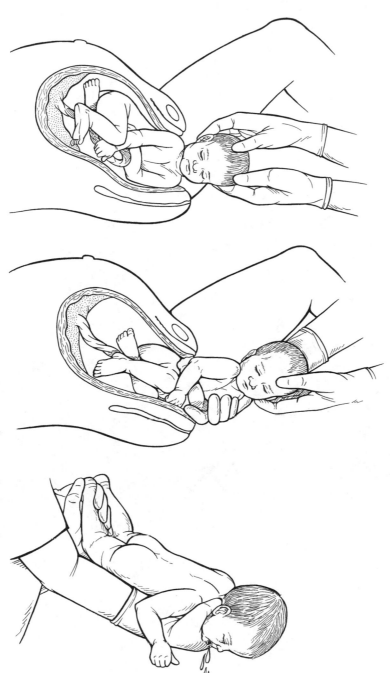

Figure 27-1:
Support the baby's head with your hands. As the rest of the body comes out, move one hand under the shoulder area. Finally, hold the baby on his or her stomach to let the fluids drain from the mouth.

Chapter 28

Special Needs of the Disabled

Statistics tell us that one out of every six people in the United States is affected by a disability. By definition, a disability limits or destroys the body's ability to accomplish certain functions. Birth defects, heredity, illness, and injury are just a few of the causes behind them.

But while the term disability can be defined, the people who have them can't be generalized. Each individual has unique abilities — and unique needs — so caring for such a person in the event of an emergency can be a challenge. For that reason, if you live or spend time with someone with a disability, think now about first aid and what you need to know if an accident or injury occurs.

Know the Disability

The best action you can take if you're close to a person with a disability — or if you have one yourself — is to find out as much about the condition as you can. You'll want to know:

- **Current physical state:** Find out how the person is faring day to day and what his or her abilities, limitations, and needs are.

- **Medical history:** With the person's permission, of course, look at past medical records. Ask about when the disability began, if it's progressed, and how needs have changed through the years.

- **What science has to say:** A great deal of medical research has been done on common disabling conditions, and it pays to find out what that research says. You'll find out the nature of the disability, what caused it, how it's expected to progress, and what treatments or aids are available to deal with it.

To get information on a condition, start at your local library (or a local hospital library), or ask your doctor for more resources. The World Wide Web also contains a great deal of health information and offers access to chat rooms and support groups on various types of disability.

Now, you're not trying to find out all of this information just to be nosy. If you're an expert in the disease, you'll know how best to handle any problems that arise. You'll also be able to watch out for any particular types of injuries a person may be prone to — for example, if a person has lost the sense of touch, unintentional burns may be an issue. Finally, you'll be able to ensure that the person gets the proper medical attention if it is needed. For a person with disabilities, the truth is as simple as this: Knowledge means independence.

If You're Providing First Aid . . .

Helping someone with a disability involves all the same key ingredients as helping a child, an elderly person, or a healthy adult. You should begin by asking the person if you can help — that is, ask for consent. Introduce yourself and find out what you can about how the emergency or accident happened. At all times, of course, treat the person with respect.

If you're calling for help, be sure to mention the person's disability to emergency medical services (EMS). They may need to take the information into account when providing treatment.

As you go along, explain what you are going to do *before* you do it. Show the person the bandage you're going to apply or the syringe you're using to clean out the wound. If you're uncertain whether a disability will interfere with first aid, just ask. The person will most likely tell you what you need to know.

That having been said, communication is an issue for some people with disabilities because of a disability affecting speech or mental processes.

Take stroke, for example. The brain damage that stroke leaves behind may cause *aphasia* — difficulty speaking or understanding speech. A person with that condition would have trouble expressing themselves if an emergency occurred. You, as the first-aid provider, wouldn't be able to ask questions or get answers, which would in turn make your job harder.

In that situation, look around to see if you can find someone who knows the victim and will be able to communicate with him or her (for example, a family member who knows sign language in the case of a person who is hearing-impaired). Do your best to obtain consent. If the person can't speak, they may be able to nod approval. If the person can't hear you, you may be able to gesture sufficiently to get a go-ahead. *Remember:* If the person denies your help, you should not render first aid.

As you give first aid to the person, remain calm. Keep the person informed about what you're going to do next, and ask permission if appropriate — for example, if you need to remove a leg brace to treat a wound.

What to Watch Out For

As was said, every disability is different, and every person with a disability is unique. The person's health, physical abilities, and environment all play a role in what safety issues may arise. Here is just a sampling to consider.

Falls

Many types of physical disabilities involve difficulty getting around, which makes falling a concern with those who must deal with them. To minimize problems, look over the environment with an eye for obstacles. Are there stairs to an upper level? Are door jambs raised? Is furniture arranged so the person must zigzag through the room to get to the bathroom? Take steps to make mobility a nonissue.

Medical equipment also plays a role in falls. Make sure all aids are in good repair and up-to-date. Check their safety features, as well — crutches and canes should have rubber stops to prevent slippage, and wheelchairs and the like should have reliable brakes. Also see that the person is well-equipped with any necessary enabling and assistive devices. New products are always coming on the market that may save steps — and falls.

Don't hesitate to seek medical care after a fall if necessary.

Burns

The inability to feel is a component of many kinds of disability. It contributes to an increased risk of burns because it negates the body's reflexes. A person without the ability to feel won't pull away automatically when he or she touches something hot, so a serious burn may occur before the person even realizes the situation.

To prevent burns in the kitchen, try to remove risks. Cookware should have insulated handles, and the stove should have indicators to show when the burners are hot. See Chapter 10 for more on burns and burn safety.

Infection

Infection is another risk that comes along with disability. Circulation is one factor; if blood isn't pumping fast enough, wounds won't heal quickly and may become infected or even gangrenous. Another is, again, inability to feel. A person with no sense of touch might not notice a cut or other injury right away, giving infection a chance to set in.

People who are at increased risk of infection should check the body regularly to make sure everything is in good order. Pay special attention to the bottom of the feet, looking at them with a mirror if necessary. It's easy to step on a sharp rock or thumbtack and not realize it until much later.

Also, seek medical attention if infection is suspected. If an infection isn't treated promptly, it can lead to serious complications — even amputation — in some instances.

Sudden illness

Some disabilities leave a person prone to sudden illness. Epilepsy, for example, may mean seizures. A weakened heart may mean a person is prone to cardiac arrest. Again, every person is different and has his or her own strengths and weaknesses. The key is to know what they are before emergency strikes and prepare.

Temperature regulation

Spinal cord injuries and other disabilities may leave a person without certain functions that regulate temperature. For example, a person might not be able to sweat, making it hard for the body to release excess heat. Another person might not be able to shiver, making cool temperatures a problem.

Here's an instance where knowing the person's condition comes in handy. If you realize hot or cold temps pose a problem, you can prevent hypothermia or heat-related illness by getting the person to a regulated environment.

Other safety concerns

Certain disabilities may interfere with the victim's ability to react to certain situations. For example, a person who is hearing-impaired wouldn't know if a fire alarm sounded. A person who is blind might not be able to find the closest exit in an emergency without assistance. If a person can't speak, it would be hard to call for help after an accident. Take these special needs into account if you're dealing with someone with a disability. Products are available to fill special needs — fire alarms can be equipped with flashing lights, emergency exits may have alarms that sound, and personal call buttons are available for those who might need help getting help. Ask your health care practitioner about details.

Chapter 29

Special Needs of High-Tech Workers

· ·

In This Chapter

▶ Common conditions

▶ Occupational health

· ·

*Y*ou're not a construction worker stepping from I-beam to I-beam. You're not an safari guide, showing travelers the African lion up-close and personal. Instead, you sit in front of a computer or work on an assembly line all day when you're on the job. What could go wrong in that environment? The answer, of course, is plenty.

Health on the Job

Here's a look at some common conditions that may occur on the job and what you can do to stop them in their tracks — before they stop you.

Allergies and other reactions

In the workplace, you'll find plenty of substances that could trigger an allergic reaction, skin condition, or worse. These substances include anything from industrial chemicals such as formaldehyde to more commonly used materials such as toner or turpentine. If you're sensitive to the substance, you may face an allergic reaction (see Chapter 19) or possibly poisoning (see Chapter 12).

If you come in contact with a harmful substance, follow your employer's guidelines on how to handle it. Federal regulations state that you have the right to know what hazardous substances you're handling in the workplace, and your employer should have that information available to you. Just ask to see the Material Safety Data Sheets (or MSDS), which supply information regarding the products you may come in contact with.

Another tip is to wash your hands frequently to remove any contaminants from the skin *before* they linger long enough to cause a reaction. Also remember to wear protective clothing. To prevent accidents, store chemicals and solvents properly and put them away when you've finished using them.

Backache

Whether you're on your feet all day or plopped behind a desk, backache may be an issue for you. You see, the spinal cord is a highly sophisticated bit of anatomy, and too much pressure, twisting, or even being still for too long can throw a wrench into its works.

While the workplace offers some risks for backache, you can mitigate them by knowing the steps to prevention:

- ✔ Don't twist and bend to get files while you're sitting down. Get out of your chair and squat down instead.

- ✔ Don't squish the phone between your ear and shoulder. Get a phone rest that attaches to the receiver so it can be held comfortably. Other options include a speakerphone or headset phone.

- ✔ Make sure you're at the right angle. Most desks aren't at the right height for reading and writing, but you can adjust them with a slant board, an angled surface available in art and drafting supply stores.

- ✔ Adjust your computer screen correctly. The National Institute for Occupational Safety and Health (NIOSH) dictates that a computer keyboard should be placed 26 to 28 inches from the floor (the average desk is 30 to 32 inches high), and the screen should be angled so that the top of the screen is 10 degrees below eye level.

What should you do if a minor backache strikes? First, stop whatever it is you're doing and sit or lie in a comfortable position. If you feel up to it, try some gentle stretching: Stand up, put your hands on your hips, and lean slowly backward, or lie on your back and pull each knee up to your chest one at a time.

Apply an ice pack wrapped in a towel every few hours for the first two days after the attack to help reduce swelling. Then switch to a heating pad for a few days to help begin the healing process.

While a minor, muscular backache can be helped with these self-care procedures, don't hesitate to seek medical care if you're dealing with something more serious. *Remember:* Don't move a person who has a suspected back injury. Instead, call on your emergency medical system (EMS) for assistance.

Carpal tunnel syndrome

Carpal tunnel is the grand master of repetitive motion injuries — injuries that occur after doing the same gesture over and over again. Carpal tunnel often affects secretaries, writers, and programmers because of typing involved in their jobs, but it also strikes industrial workers who must keep up with the assembly line.

In carpal tunnel syndrome, the tendons in the fingers become swollen, putting pressure on the main nerve in the wrist. Slightly more than one-third of people with jobs requiring repetitive movements get carpal tunnel syndrome, and about one-third of those who have it get it in both wrists at the same time.

With carpal tunnel, pain occurs in the palm, thumb, and index and middle fingers, and possibly in the wrist and forearm. A tingling sensation when you tap the wrist on the skin creases on the palm side is also a sign.

Carpal tunnel sets in slowly, but if you suspect you have it, visit a physician. In the meantime, try keeping your wrist above the level of your elbow to relieve pressure on the nerve. And, of course, vary your routine as much as possible. Take short breaks from typing or whatever activity is triggering the condition. Or switch off with a coworker who has a different sort of motion to perform.

Another tip is to get yourself a padded wrist support for your computer keyboard. The long, narrow pad lies just below the keyboard and helps keep your hands and wrist at a proper angle to prevent carpal tunnel. Mousepad versions of this aid are also now available.

If the condition is minor, switching your routine, wearing a simple wrist brace, and avoiding repetitive motion may resolve it. Treatment for more severe cases includes wearing a wrist brace, getting cortisone injections, and having surgery.

Eye strain

Looking at a computer screen all day isn't like reading. Instead of deciphering ink on a page, you're essentially interpreting different colors and shades of light. And that can get pretty hard on the eyes, resulting in a condition called eye strain.

Symptoms of eye strain include dry eyes, tired eyes, and headache. To help prevent the condition, take regular, short breaks from your work, even if it's just a few minutes for a trip to the water fountain. Plan your day so that your computer time is broken up by other tasks, such as opening mail or attending a meeting.

Also follow the guidelines from the National Institute for Occupational Safety and Health, mentioned earlier. Again, they say that a computer keyboard should be placed 26 to 28 inches from the floor (the average desk is 30 to 32 inches high), and the screen should be angled so that the top of the screen is 10 degrees below eye level.

If eye strain persists, see your eye doctor for treatment. Over-the-counter pain relievers or eye drops may help temporarily, but you'll want to get your eyes checked and glasses adjusted if needed. Another solution, of course, is cutting back your time in front of the TV or computer.

Occupational hazards

Occupational health is a discipline that deals with a person's safety and physical well-being on the job. The National Institute for Occupational Safety and Health is the government organization devoted to preventing problems in the workplace. For more information on occupational hazards, write to NIOSH at Robert A. Taft Laboratories, 4676 Columbia Parkway, MS C-19, Cincinnati, OH 45226-1998.

Part VI
The Part of Tens

The 5th Wave

By Rich Tennant

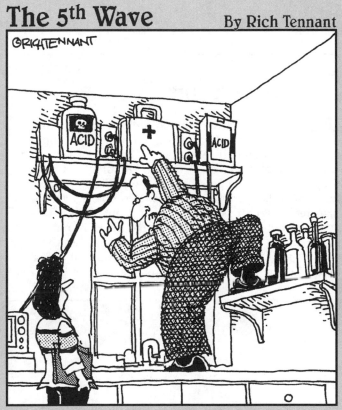

"We keep the first-aid kit where it's handy, but out of the children's reach. Just step into the sink and then brace your other foot on this shelf where we keep the cooking oil. It's right up here next to the electrical sockets and acid."

In this part . . .

How do you get the most information across in the least number of pages? *...For Dummies* has figured it out with their signature format of The Part of Tens. Just check through these quick lists to find plenty of helpful tips and truths that support and supplement your first-aid fundamentals. Want to know how to prepare for a natural disaster? Read on. Need help picking out an over-the-counter medication? You've come to the right place. Investigating natural remedies for your ills? Get the scoop in these pages. Searching for more info on first aid or health in general? Look no further. It's all right here.

Chapter 30

Ten Ways to Prepare for an Emergency

Tornadoes, hurricanes, earthquakes, floods, chemical spills, and fires threaten somewhere in the United States practically every day. In the event a disaster occurs, first aid is among the most valuable skills you can have. But first aid is just one of the things that you need to know. In this chapter, you'll find ten other tips to keeping you and your family safe if disaster strikes.

Plan Your Plan

You know that it's important to have an evacuation plan should your house catch on fire, but did you know that you should also plan now for a possible disaster? Take some time to think about what problems might occur in your area. Is your region prone to tornadoes? Do you live near a river that may flood? Have hurricanes been known to blow through town? Pick the most likely problems and find out the best course of action to take in each of them. Talk about possible evacuation routes and where you might go if you couldn't stay in your home.

Settle Your Supplies

In addition to your first-aid kit, you should set aside a supply of nonperishable foods — dry or canned foods that won't spoil without refrigeration — just in case of an emergency. Store enough for each member of your family (including any pets) to last a few days. You'll need to set aside one gallon of water per person, per day, for drinking, as well as another quart or two for each for personal uses. Keep the water in plastic, not glass, bottles to prevent accidents with broken glass.

What types of food should you store? Choose a selection of canned fruits and vegetables, as well as canned meats, nuts, and peanut butter (which are high in protein). Try to pick foods that won't need cooking or preparation. And don't forget the can opener!

Once the food and water is out of the way, think about other items you might need, such as a flashlight, a spare set of car keys, batteries, blankets, a change of clothes, or a deck of cards. Also consider any special items, such as prescription medications, eyeglasses, or diapers and formula for an infant.

This is also the time to get your personal papers in order. Copies of pertinent financial statements, insurance policies, and medical records should be made and safely stored. It's also a good idea to make a list of valuable items in your home and photograph or videotape them "for the record." Make sure you note serial numbers and model numbers. Store your notes in a safe place — perhaps even in a safe deposit box or another spot away from your home.

Allow for Communication

In a disaster, you need to act and react to keep you and your family safe. And to do that effectively, you need to know what's going on at all times. For that reason, keep a radio with fresh batteries on hand at all times — and know what stations broadcast instructions if there is an emergency. Emergency broadcasts are also available on certain television stations (think of that rainbow test pattern and the reassuring voice saying, "This is a test, this is only a test"). Another option is a special emergency radio, available from the National Weather Service, that sounds an alarm when bad weather is predicted.

Help Out Your Home

The better condition your home is in *before* disaster strikes, the better it will fare when push comes to shove. Repair cracks in the walls or any loose wiring — defective electrical wiring may cause fire. Also fasten in place any furniture that may fall or break in a disaster — items like tall bookshelves, large paintings, mirrors, or light fixtures. You should know where your gas and electric cut-off switches are in case they're needed.

Care for Your Car

If you need to leave your home behind in the event of an emergency, your car may be essential. Keep it in good repair and do your best to keep at least a half-tank of gas at all times (a tip that's handy in general, not just in an emergency). Stow a first-aid kit in the back (see Chapter 4 for a list of the contents), and make sure you have other essentials: jumper cables, flares, flashlight, and so on, on hand. An emergency stash of nonperishable foods, a few blankets, and other disaster supplies (already discussed earlier in this chapter) should also be prepared.

Think About Others

While you may tend to focus on your immediate family when preparing for the worst, don't forget about the others in your life. Talk to grandparents and other relatives, as well as your neighbors, about what they'll do if disaster strikes. You may want to include them somehow in your disaster plan. For example, if an elderly person lives nearby, you may make a note to call their children if a problem arises or even make plans to help them evacuate if necessary.

Consider Special Needs

People with specific medical conditions and disabilities, the elderly, and even children all have special needs that must be taken into account when preparing for disaster. If you're setting aside supplies, make sure you have everything needed. A person with a wheelchair, for example, might need an extra battery. A baby would need diapers and formula. A person with diabetes would need a good supply of insulin. And even a person with glasses would need a spare pair (or at least a copy of the prescription). Take these issues into consideration when planning.

Prepare Your Pets

When you're planning for an emergency or stocking up on canned goods, it's easy to forget you need to allow for your pets, too. Make sure to set aside food and water, a secure carrier or leash, medical records and other information, and any easy-to-transport toys for your pet. Also decide what you'll do if you can't take your pet with you — if you need to go to an emergency shelter, for example, your pet won't be allowed. If that happens, you may need to put up your pet in a motel that accept pets, a kennel or veterinarians office, or a friend's or relative's house. Don't leave your pet behind!

Do the Right Thing

If an emergency or disaster occurs, your local officials will tell you if and when you need to leave your home. If they tell you to leave pronto, don't stop to fuss about your house. Just take your disaster supplies that you've already set aside and get out of the area. However, if you have time to prepare (for example, if a hurricane or flood is expected to hit in a few days), action can be taken to help minimize damage.

Your house will be better off if you take some time to look for potential problems. Bring your outdoor equipment and furniture inside, and "batten down" any structures that might be damaged or swept away (such as air conditioning units, propane tanks, and the like). Inside your home, move your belongings so they're away from windows or, in the case of flooding, they're on upper floors of the house.

To protect your windows in high winds, cover them with plywood or shutters so they're not shattered by flying debris. Stretching tape across windows is another step many people take, but be warned that it doesn't deter breakage — it just prevents the broken glass from getting all over the place.

If flooding is expected, sandbags may be used to protect your home from water. According to the American Red Cross, it takes two people one hour to fill and place 100 bags, which will make you a wall 1 foot high and 20 feet long. If you try sandbags, just make sure you have enough manpower and time to do it properly.

Finally, turn off your electricity, water, and propane service (if you use one). Don't, however, turn off natural gas because it will require a professional to turn it back on again.

Review Your Plan Regularly

Once you're all set for a potential disaster, don't just forget about your plan. Review it regularly to see if anything has changed. Construction and development may alter evacuation routes, for example, or a neighbor you're depending on might move. Double-check your supplies and first-aid kit, too, to make sure items haven't gone beyond their expiration dates and can still be used. Food and water supplies should be replaced every six months.

Chapter 31

Ten OTC Products for Self-Care

*T*he first-aid kit is different from the medicine cabinet, but the medicine cabinet and the over-the-counter (OTC) medications it holds are still an arsenal in the face of an emergency.

OTCs are medications you can buy in drugstores, supermarkets, and department stores without a doctor's prescription. OTCs are rigorously tested by the U.S. Food and Drug Administration and are generally safe for use by most people when the manufacturer's instructions (printed on the label) are followed. In addition, they're affordable and convenient, and give people a measure of control over their own health.

With between 125,000 and 300,000 over-the-counter drugs on the market today, stocking your medicine cabinet can be a daunting feat. This chapter narrows down the field by suggesting ten categories of OTCs that are helpful during or after an emergency — or just essential to have on hand. To help you track down a product on your own, the generic name of the drug has been followed by the brand name in parentheses (if there is a brand name).

As you read these pages, you'll find warnings and tips about each medication. However, you must remember that all drugs — even OTC drugs — are powerful substances that can alter the body. If they're taken incorrectly, they may cause damage. Likewise, if a person is allergic or sensitive to a drug, it may cause side effects. Another risk: Certain medications taken in combination can react with each other (or even with food or vitamins) to cause harm. For all of these reasons, use OTC drugs only according to manufacturer's instructions and always keep your health care provider and pharmacist up to date on all the medications you're taking.

Nonsteroidal Anti-inflammatory Drugs (NSAIDs)

Whether you have a cut on your hand, a sore on your foot, or an ache in your head, chances are you'll turn to your medicine cabinet — and a nonsteroidal anti-inflammatory drug — for relief.

Nonsteroidal anti-inflammatory drugs, called NSAIDs, sound like heavy duty drugs, if the length of the name is any indication. However, they are among the most common and best OTC drugs for pain and fever relief. By blocking the production of inflammatory chemicals called prostaglandins at the site of an injury, NSAIDs help ease stiffness and inflammation. In addition, they're often taken to help prevent heart and circulatory problems.

Ibuprofen (Advil, Motrin IB, Nuprin), naproxen (Aleve, Naprosyn), and keto-profen (Actron, Orudis) are three types of NSAIDs on the market today. Ibuprofen is the most easily found NSAID, while naproxen offers the longest relief (eight hours, as compared with four or six with other products).

Aspirin (Anacin, Bayer, Bufferin, Ecotrin) is also an NSAID, although it carries the risk of greater stomach irritation than others in its family. It's also not recommended for children under 21 years of age because it has been linked to Reye's syndrome, a potentially fatal brain and liver disorder.

Acetaminophen is a related product, often called "nonaspirin" on the label. Like NSAIDs, acetaminophen helps relieve pain and fever. However, it doesn't help in the inflammation department. That's because it works in the brain to ease the perception of pain — rather than halts the production of prostaglandins triggered by injury. Still, acetaminophen might be the choice for people with sensitive stomachs because it doesn't cause upset stomachs or bleeding problems like aspirin might. It's also the safest choice for pregnant women and is recommended for children under 21 years (see Reye's warning). Acetaminophen is sold under the brand names Anacin, Bayer, Excedrin, and Tylenol, just to name a few.

Antiseptics

If the word *antiseptic* sounds to you a little like *disinfectant,* that's no coincidence. Both products do the same thing — that is, prevent the growth of microorganisms. Antiseptics are used on the skin after a burn or cut to cleanse the area and prevent infection. Disinfectants, on the other hand, are stronger than antiseptics and not recommended for the skin. Instead, use them on your countertops.

Most antiseptics come in liquid form and include hydrogen peroxide, alcohol, isopropyl alcohol, and iodine. They are all good at killing germs, but each has its own characteristics. For example, because hydrogen peroxide works through the chemical release of oxygen, it shouldn't be used on abscesses or unbroken skin and should be allowed to dry before the area is bandaged. Alcohol and isopropyl alcohol (which is the stronger of the two) may dry the skin. And iodine tends to irritate skin and so shouldn't be used with a bandage. In some people it causes allergic reaction.

Antibiotics

Antibiotics are prescription drugs, usually taken orally to help drive out infections like strep throat. But in their OTC form, antibiotics are more likely used to help prevent infection in minor cuts and scrapes. They're applied right to the skin, as creams and ointments, not taken by mouth.

Common antibiotics include bacitracin (Bacitracin) and neomycin (Clomycin, Mycitracin, Neosporin). A product that combines bacitracin with another antibiotic, called polymyxin B sulfate (Polysporin), is especially recommended because it's effective against many different types of infection. Neomycin tends to cause an allergic reaction in 5 to 8 percent of the people who use it.

Astringents

Astringents work by coagulating the protein in skin cells. While it doesn't sound like an impressive job, the protective skin coating that coagulation leaves behind reduces swelling and aids healing. They can be used on their own on a dressing or compress, but they're also often found in other OTC products that treat problems such as hemorrhoids and insect bites and stings.

Aluminum acetate (Burow's solution), witch hazel, and zinc oxide and calamine (Gold Bond, Calamine) are astringents you're likely to find on drugstore shelves. Aluminum acetate will need to be diluted according to package instructions, but witch hazel can be applied right to the skin. The mildest of the three, zinc oxide and calamine are thought to be good for diaper rash.

Topical Antihistamines

To understand antihistamines, you first need to know a little about how the body works. When you come in contact with a substance that you're sensitive or allergic to, the production of chemicals called histamines begins in response. Histamines, in turn, cause blood vessels to enlarge and swell — a reaction recognized as a hive or rash.

Antihistamines, as the name suggests, fight histamines to reduce swelling and throw in a little numbing action at the same time. They're helpful when dealing with minor burns and cuts, sunburn, insect bites, and other little irritations. They come in cream, spray, and gel forms, and common types include diphenhydramine (Benadryl Itch Stopping Cream/Spray/Gel), triplennamine, and pyrilamine. An antihistamine shouldn't be used regularly for more than a week at a time. In some people, the antihistamine itself causes an allergic reaction.

What about oral antihistamines (Actifed, Benadryl, Sudafed)? While they're usually used to treat coughs and colds, they work the same way as topical antihistamines do — by combating histamines. For that reason, they still have a first-aid use: They can be taken to relieve itching on a whole-body level and may help a person sleep more easily despite hives or a rash.

Hydrocortisone

Hydrocortisone (Bactine, Cortaid, Cortizone-5) is closely related to antihistamine. But while an antihistamine competes with the chemicals that cause an allergic reaction, hydrocortisone stops them before they can even be produced. In its topical form, hydrocortisone is used for minor skin irritations, itching, and rashes, including those caused by poisonous plants and irritating household products. It's especially good for itchiness caused by dry skin conditions like eczema. However, if you're dealing with an allergic reaction, an antihistamine is the better bet because it relieves symptoms faster. On the other hand, antihistamines themselves carry a small risk of allergic reaction, while hydrocortisone is much milder.

Antacids

Antacids are, admittedly, not a front-line weapon in the first-aider's war against accident or injury, but who has ever heard of a medicine cabinet without them? Used to relieve heartburn, indigestion, and other aches and pains in the stomach, the antacid is about as standard (and necessary) an OTC as you can get.

Most traditional antacids work by combining with stomach acids and turning them into harmless salt and water. However, a number of newer antacids have been created that inhibit the production of stomach acid even before it starts. That means that you can prevent indigestion before the first symptoms set in.

Traditional antacids — the ones that work with stomach acid — include sodium bicarbonate (Alka-Seltzer), calcium carbonate (Maalox, Mylanta, Rolaids, Tums), and aluminum and magnesium (Di-Gel, Gaviscon). New, preventative antacids are cimetidine (Tagamet HB), ranitidine (Zantac 75), and famotidine (Pepcid AC).

One exception to the whole scheme is bismuth subsalicylate (Pepto-Bismol). It doesn't work like either of its sister antacids. Instead, it lessens stomach aches by suppressing Helicobacter pylori, stomach-dwelling germs that are thought responsible for inflammation. One word of warning here: This OTC contains salicylates, which have been linked to Reye's disease in children under age 21. Reye's disease is a potentially fatal brain and liver disorder.

Don't know which antacid to stock up on? Traditional antacids generally work quickly and provide adequate relief of symptoms. But if you know you're in for a rough evening (say, if chili dogs are in the menu), the new generation may be a better choice.

Emetics

Emetics are OTC remedies that induce vomiting. They're used primarily in poisoning emergencies to rid the system of the toxic substance.

Even though an emetic is something to have on hand, it's not something that you should ever readily use. In fact, never use an emetic without direction from a physician or the poison control center. The reason is this: If the poison that was ingested is caustic, it'll do more damage to the stomach, esophagus, and mouth if it's brought back up than if it's neutralized somehow within the body.

You have two types of emetics to choose from: syrup of ipecac and activated charcoal. Syrup of ipecac irritates the lining of the stomach while it triggers an area of the brain linked to vomiting. Follow the poison control center's and manufacturer's instructions, and be careful with the dosage — too much will cause repeated vomiting and serious heart problems.

Activated charcoal is your other option. It's mixed with water and then swallowed down into the digestive system, where it absorbs poisons in the system. Both methods work equally well, but the decision of which to use depends on the direction you'll get from poison control or a health care provider. In addition, ipecac may be a better option for children, who don't like the ugly taste of a charcoal slurry. And another warning: Don't use charcoal and ipecac together — the charcoal will simply absorb the ipecac and both substances will be rendered useless.

Counterirritants

Ever heard the joke about the sadist's cure for a headache? Step on your foot. Surprisingly, the principle behind counterirritants, OTCs used to reduce pain from sprained or strained muscles, is remarkably similar.

These OTC drugs produce irritation and minor pain in nearby tissues, giving relief from the more intense pain the injury is causing. No one is quite sure how this works. It might be because the irritation resulted in increased blood flow, raising skin temperature. Another theory is that all nerve impulses regarding pain are passed through the same area of the spinal cord, so the sensation of irritation takes away from the more intense pain.

Counterirritants come in handy in the days and weeks after an injury has occurred. They are usually sold as creams and ointments that can be rubbed on the affected area, although liquid forms are also available. Specific products include oil of wintergreen (Ben Gay, Exocaine), camphor, menthol (Asorbine Jr., Therapeutic Mineral Ice), capsicum (Capzasin-P, Zostrix), and trolamine salicylate (Aspercreme, Sportscreme). Ask your doctor about the best choice for your particular injury.

Antidiarrheals

This medicine cabinet staple, as the name implies, helps to relieve diarrhea that's not caused by a specific condition such as food poisoning or infection.

If there's a chance that diarrhea is caused by an infection or food poisoning (which comes from eating undercooked or contaminated food), don't self-treat. Instead, seek medical care.

Antidiarrheals come in three different forms. Loperamide (Imodium A-D, Kaopectate 1-D) is the most common *antiperistaltic* drug. It works by slowing the rate at which fecal matter passes through the intestines, and it works best on mild diarrhea. Attapulgite (Diasorb, Kaopectate, Rheaban) is a common *adsorbent,* a medication that binds with the material in the digestive system to harden stool. It is most effective for sudden, more severe diarrhea. *Bismuth subsalicylate* (Pepto-Bismol) is the third form, and it works by inhibiting the organisms that cause diarrhea. It's the only form of antidiarrheal that can prevent, as well as treat, the condition.

Chapter 32

Ten Things to Know about Natural Remedies

A hundred years ago, you couldn't just walk into a drugstore or supermarket to pick up Pepto-Bismol or antibacterial ointment. Instead, you would have relied on natural remedies whose recipes had been handed down from generation to generation. While the traditional medical world has made great strides and advancements since those days, natural remedies still hold their place in the treatment of illness and disease. In fact, they're becoming more and more popular — and available — in today's society.

Why the resurgence of popularity for natural remedies? For one thing, they tend to be less expensive than traditional drugs. For another, they tend to have fewer side effects. But that doesn't mean that natural remedies are for everyone, or that they're for every situation. This chapter provides an introduction to natural remedies and what you need to know to use them safely and effectively.

Know Your Options

Natural remedies fall into the realm of complementary medicine: the label given to therapies that aren't considered traditional medicine in the United States. Complementary medicine includes everything from acupuncture and acupressure to sound therapy and biofeedback. At one time, these therapies were termed *alternative* therapies because they were alternatives to so-called regular medical care. However, the term *complementary* is now frequently used as a testament to the fact that these practices may be used *along with* traditional medicine to benefit the patient.

For the purposes of first aid, the scope of complementary medicine can be narrowed to include a few key categories.

Herbalism

Thousands of years ago, plants were the first medicines. In fact, many experts speculate that ancient people observed the plants that sick animals ate and then tried them out themselves when they were under the weather. Today, this tradition continues. Herbs, which come in many different forms (and are applied in many different ways), are used to treat a wide range of conditions, from allergies to menopause.

Herbs can be quite powerful, so it's recommended that you get professional advice on how to use them correctly. Herbs have been known to trigger heart attacks, miscarriage and early labor, and severe allergic reactions.

Homeopathy

Homeopathy uses safe, natural substances to stimulate the body's healing processes. It is based on the theory that "like cures like" — that what creates symptoms in a healthy person will cure a sick person with the same symptoms. Remedies are available in liquid or tablet form and are taken by mouth. Because homeopathic substances are almost completely diluted, they have no side effects.

Bach flower essences

These remedies are made by soaking flower blossoms and other organic material in a mixture of water and alcohol. Those who use the essences maintain that they affect mood and the body's natural energy and promote good health. The mixtures, available in health food stores, are nontoxic and have no side effects.

Acupressure

This Chinese therapy is based on a belief in a life force called *chi,* which is thought to flow throughout the body along 12 major pathways called *meridians.* According to traditional Chinese thinking, if your *chi* is flowing smoothly, you feel emotionally and physically healthy. However, if your *chi* is out of whack, illness will result.

Acupressure helps to correct the flow of *chi* by stimulating specific spots (called pressure points) with the fingers or a wooden dowel. The pressure is thought to restore the flow of *chi*. Acupressure can be practiced in the home and has no side effects. However, it should be avoided if a person is pregnant or seriously ill. Also avoid touching areas that are burned, injured, or infected.

Massage

If you've ever submitted to a back rub to help ease your aching muscles, you've practiced this complementary therapy. Massage promotes healing by releasing physical muscle tension, improving circulation, and encouraging relaxation. It works best for minor aches and pains and conditions related to stress. Like acupressure, massage is generally safe. However, don't try it on pregnant women or the seriously ill. Avoid burned, injured, or infected areas of the body.

Aromatherapy

Aromatherapy is the use of scent to promote relaxation and to relieve symptoms and conditions. It's used for aches, allergies, arthritis, mood swings, headaches, and menstrual and menopausal symptoms, among other things.

Essential oils — concentrated plant products — form the basis of aromatherapy. These oils are diluted with water or heated to release their scents, which are thought to stimulate the brain and encourage healing and relaxation They are also sometimes applied, in diluted form, directly to the skin.

Risks of essential oils are few, though they've been known to cause allergic reactions in sensitive people. People who are pregnant or have a history of seizures and high blood pressure should consult a professional before using essential oils. In their pure form, essential oils should be kept out of reach of children.

A host of other folklore and remedies exist that don't fall into any of these categories — for example, the art of washing your warts in stump water to make them disappear. While you probably don't want to rely on recipes like this to preserve your family's health, it's worth pointing out that a few of these natural remedies do have value. Oranges, for example, were once the folk remedy for scurvy (now known to be treated with vitamin C). Baking soda makes a good treatment for heartburn. Even simple cold water does wonders to stop the progression of a burn.

Know When Not to Use Natural Remedies

Now that you know a little about what remedies are helpful in first aid situations, recognize the best situations in which to use them. Some natural remedies are excellent as first aid, but sometimes there's just no substitute for professional medical care.

If you're dealing with a serious circumstance, such as a broken bone, head injury, internal bleeding, choking, or heart or breathing problem, stick with the tried-and-true first-aid techniques discussed in this book and call for emergency medical services (EMS) when appropriate.

Natural remedies are more appropriate for minor, non–life-threatening problems, such as insect bites, small cuts and bruises, rashes, fevers, and stomach discomforts. But here, too, use your best judgment and seek medical care if it becomes necessary. A prolonged fever in a child, for example, calls for a doctor's care, and even a minor cut may become infected. If you're in doubt as to whether to call in a medical professional, err on the side of caution and do it. Better to be safe than sorry.

Understand That "Natural" Doesn't Mean "Harmless"

Cheerleaders for natural remedies argue, rightly, that herbs and homeopathy and the like have fewer side effects than over-the-counter drugs. But just because they're natural, don't think they're completely harmless. Certain herbs can trigger heart attack and high blood pressure — even miscarriage. Other remedies may cause allergic reactions in sensitive people. With this in mind, follow instructions when using natural remedies and consult your physician or a complementary practitioner when in doubt. Just like prescription medications, natural remedies should be treated with respect.

Do Your Homework

Don't expect to learn everything you need to know about natural remedies by reading the labels of products in the health food store. To really understand your options and the capabilities of different therapies, you need to do some research. Your local library likely has a host of books on the more popular complementary therapies, such as herbalism. Some books focus specifically on using natural remedies for first aid. You can also look in the phone book to hook up with those in your community that practice complementary medicine.

Don't forget about cyberspace when you're doing your research — just be sure to take what your find with a grain of salt. You'll find a multitude of "junk" sites out there touting "Joe's Miracle Rocks" and other nonsense remedies, so don't just act on what you see. Look for reputable sites, like the National Institutes of Health's National Center for Complementary and Alternative Medicine Clearinghouse site, found at `http://nccam.nih.gov/nccam/clearinghouse/`.

Complementary therapies aren't standardized, so different texts and individuals may offer different advice on using remedies. That's to be expected with such an inexact science, but be careful to use reputable sources when looking for treatments on your own. If possible, seek out a licensed or certified practitioner of the healing art you're interested in.

Learn the Lingo

As you're researching natural remedies, you'll come across a number of terms that might be unfamiliar, especially when it comes to herbalism. Here are just a few of the words you might come across:

- **Compress:** A piece of clean cloth or gauze soaked in an herbal preparation such as an infusion or decoction. The compress is then applied directly to the skin.

- **Infusion:** An herbal preparation in which the herb is steeped in hot water.

- **Decoction:** An herbal preparation in which the herb is boiled. Decoctions are used for woody herbs such as roots and barks.

- **Liniment:** A mixture of alcohol and herbal oils that, when rubbed on the muscles, improves circulation.

- **Poultice:** An application of an herb directly to the skin. The herb may first be dried or crushed and mixed with water to create a paste. The herb is then covered with a bandage to hold it in place.

- **Tincture:** An herbal preparation in which the herb is steeped in a mixture of alcohol and water for several weeks. Tinctures are often available already prepared.

Keep Your Doctor Informed

Remember, complementary therapies are just that: complementary. They're intended to be used along with traditional medical care when necessary to benefit the health of a patient. To this end, keep your regular doctor up to date on what natural remedies you're using, whether it's colloidal oatmeal in a bath to soothe a rash or an herbal poultice to soothe a burn.

Telling your doctor the details is important for a few reasons. First of all, as you've read, not all complementary therapies are without risk, and your doctor may be able to point out a pitfall. Secondly, some natural remedies may interfere with prescription or over-the-counter medications, making them more powerful or rendering them useless. A doc can spot such problems before they happen. Your practitioner should also be kept informed so he can adjust your treatment accordingly. If you're rapidly improving because of a natural remedy, your doc needs to know.

Learn from a Pro

If you want to put natural remedies to the test, it's best to get advice from someone who knows what's what. Unfortunately, finding a practitioner of complementary medicine can be difficult in many communities, but here are a few tips to help make it a little easier:

- **Start with friends and coworkers:** Ask if anyone can refer your to someone they know.

- **Look in the phone book:** If you don't see anyone listed under the therapy you'd like to try, check under "therapeutic massage." Even if you're not into massage, there's a chance that person might be able to refer you to someone who works in the area you are interested in.

- **Talk to your doctor:** You should be keeping your doctor up-to-date on your complementary activities anyway, so tap this resource. Although many doctors are out of touch with this segment of the medical community, you may get lucky.

- **Go to the library:** Books and magazines on complementary medicine often list resources that can lead you to practitioners in your area.

- **Contact an organization:** National organizations exist for therapies such as herbalism and acupressure, and many such groups will point you in the right direction if you want to learn more.

Check Out References

Knowing who is and isn't qualified to teach you or treat you in the world of complementary medicine is a challenge. But there are two criteria to help you evaluate practitioners in certain fields:

✔ Licensing refers to state requirements that a practitioner must meet before being allowed to practice in that state. For example, a homeopathic physician in Arizona must be licensed before practicing. However, other states have no licensing requirements for homeopathy, so physicians can practice there without meeting any standards.

✔ Certification refers to the course of study a practitioner may complete to demonstrate competency. Unlike licensing, certification is not required by law in order to practice. But certification will show that a person has been trained at a specific school in a particular program, and that can help you determine whether the practitioner is qualified.

Watch Your Wallet

Despite the fact that complementary medicine is becoming more and more accepted, most are still not covered by health insurance. That means that even though complementary therapies tend to be cheaper than traditional ones, you may end up paying even more out of pocket than you would if you went right to your regular doctor. To avoid being caught with unanticipated expenses, find out the cost of a particular course of treatment *before* undergoing it. In some cases, you may be able to work out a payment plan if the price is too much for you to handle all at once.

On the brighter side, things are looking up for coverage of complementary therapies. As more becomes known about these treatments — and as they're proven to be effective — insurance companies are beginning to pick up the tab for certain procedures. Hydrotherapy and massage may be covered when used as a method of physical therapy, for example. And acupuncture, which was recently officially recognized as effective by the National Institutes of Health, may also soon be covered.

Don't Stop Here

For more information on specific therapies and natural remedies, get in touch with the following groups:

- **Herbalism:** American Botanical Council, P.O. Box 201660, Austin, TX 78720; (512) 331-8868; www.herbalgram.org

  American Herbalists Guild, P.O. Box 746555, Arvada, CO 80006; (303) 423-8800

  Association of Natural Medicine Pharmacists, 8369 Champs de Elysses, Forestville, CA 95436; (707) 887-1351

- **Homeopathy:** International Foundation for Homeopathy, P.O. Box 7, Edmonds, WA 98020; (206) 776-4147

  National Center for Homeopathy, 801 N. Fairfax St., Suite 306, Alexandria, VA 22314; (703) 548-7790; www.healthy.net/nch

- **Massage therapy:** American Massage Therapy Association, 820 Davis St., Suite 100, Evanston, IL 60201-4444; (708) 864-0123

- **Acupressure:** American Association of Acupuncture and Oriental Medicine, 433 Front St., Catasauqua, PA 18032; (610) 433-2448

Chapter 33

Ten Places to Go for More Information

*H*ealth is a hot topic these days, so you don't want to start and end with this book. In the following pages, you'll find ten helpful information resources worth knowing. While some are devoted to first-aid issues, others provide tips on safety, accident prevention, and even general health.

It's not a good idea to wait to call an organization or look up a Web site until an emergency arises. Instead, pursue these resources when all is well so that you have the information on hand (or in your head) should an accident occur. In addition, don't substitute the information found on-line, or even in this book, for medical advice. Everyone is different, and only your practitioner can diagnose and treat conditions appropriately. While the Internet is a powerful tool, it's not a doctor.

But it is a good idea to keep in mind an organization's background when checking out its information. This listing contains for-profit and nonprofit groups, and each has its own affiliations and bias. You might come across fundraising efforts, petitions, or advertisements for books — or even doctors and hospitals — but know that these sites are not on this list for any of those features, but rather because they're helpful health resources.

That having been said, here goes!

American Association of Poison Control Centers (AAPCC)

The AAPCC is a national association of poison control centers that's involved in education, prevention, and legislative matters regarding poisoning. Its Web site (www.aapcc.org) has safety tips, games, and information on recent bills and laws, but you won't find much on first aid — that's because it *isn't* the place to go if an emergency strikes. The site will, however, give you the names and contact information of poison control centers in your state, as well as poison control educators in your area. And although the association itself doesn't provide brochures and fact sheets, it will lead you to a local center that can do just that.

American Association of Retired Persons

The AARP is an organization of men and women over the age of 50 that is dedicated to enhancing the quality of life for seniors. Although nonprofit, the group is political, taking an advocacy role in many government and legislative debates. But forgive us if their beliefs don't mirror yours — the group is listed here simply because it provides health resources specifically for seniors on its Web site at www.aarp.org/indexes/health.html. The address for the group is AARP, 601 E St., N.W., Washington, DC 20049; (800) 424-3410 or (202) 434-2277.

American Heart Association (AHA)

The AHA is a nonprofit group that deals with heart disease and stroke. Consequently, it offers to the public information about cardiopulmonary resuscitation (CPR) and other emergency procedures that may be related to these conditions. Information is available on-line (www.americanheart.org), and the group also offers classes at the local level on CPR and the like. Write or call: American Heart Association, 7272 Greenville Ave., Dallas, TX 75231-4596; (800) AHA-USA1 or (214) 373-6300.

American Red Cross

Of course, the American Red Cross must be on any list of resources on first aid. After all, they (literally) wrote the book on the subject, and the organization's local chapters bring that book to life by offering courses at the community level. You can find out how to contact your chapter on the Red Cross Web site (www.redcross.org), or call (703) 248-4222. Its mailing address is American Red Cross, Attn: Public Inquiry Office, 11th floor, 1621 N. Kent Street, Arlington, VA 22209.

Burn Prevention Foundation

The Burn Prevention Foundation is a nonprofit organization devoted to teaching the public — especially children — about the dangers of fire, how to prevent it, and what to do if it occurs. The group offers educational tools and fact sheets. To contact them, write to the Burn Prevention Foundation, 5000 Tilghman Street, Suite 110, Allentown, PA 18104, or call (610) 481-9810. Their Web site, which includes a few games and plenty of tips, can be found at www.burnprevention.org.

Centers for Disease Control and Prevention (CDC)

The CDC is the prevention arm of U.S. government health projects. Their official mission is "to promote health and quality of life by preventing and controlling disease, injury, and disability." On their Web site (www.cdc.gov) look for health information in their A-Z library, check statistics, and read about recent health alerts. They also accept public calls at (404) 639-3534 or (800) 311-3435. Their address is Centers for Disease Control and Prevention, 1600 Clifton Rd., Atlanta, GA 30333.

A great resource for first aid and related information is the National Center for Injury Control and Prevention, which is part of the CDC. Its goal is to prevent deaths and injuries related to accidents in the United States by providing information, offering statistics, and running public health programs. It's Web site (www.cdc.gov/ncipc/ncipchm.htm) covers auto, bike, home safety, and much, much more. You can also write for information at National Center for Injury Prevention and Control, Mailstop K65, 4770 Buford Highway NE, Atlanta, GA 30341-3724. The phone number is (770) 488-1506.

The National Institutes for Occupational Safety and Health is also part of the CDC. It offers information about keeping your workplace healthy and safe. For information on occupational hazards, write to NIOSH at Robert A. Taft Laboratories, 4676 Columbia Parkway, MS C-19, Cincinnati, OH 45226-1998, or call (800) 35-NIOSH.

National Institutes of Health (NIH)

The National Institutes of Health is a government organization with the goal of "acquiring new knowledge to help prevent, detect, diagnose, and treat disease and disability, from the rarest genetic disorder to the common cold." Located in Bethesda, MD, the NIH is comprised of 25 different institutes and centers. Consumer information can be found on the NIH Web site (www.nih.gov), but you can also request resources directly from its specific institutes.

For example, the National Institute on Aging provides outstanding resources on dealing with health issues surrounding aging. To request materials, call (800) 222-2225 or (800) 222-4225 (hearing-impaired) between 8:30 a.m. and 5:00 p.m., Eastern Standard Time. You can also write to the NIA Information Center at P.O. Box 8057, Gaithersburg, MD 20898-8057. The NIA Web site is www.nih.gov/nia, and they also offer the "Age Pages," a special resource for seniors, at www.aoa.dhhs.gov/elderpage.html#ap.

Another branch of the NIH is the National Arthritis and Musculoskeletal and Skin Diseases Information Clearinghouse (quite a mouthful!), which can offer information on bone and joint injuries as well as arthritis and other chronic conditions. Its address is National Arthritis and Musculoskeletal and Skin Diseases Information Clearinghouse, National Institutes of Health, 1 AMS Circle, Bethesda, MD 20892-3675. The phone number is (301) 495-4484 or (301) 565-2966 (hearing-impaired). Web site? Check out www.nih.gov/niams.

Wondering whether an herbal first-aid remedy is worth trying? The National Center for Complementary and Alternative Medicine Clearinghouse is also offered by the NIH. This organization provides information to the public about complementary and alternative medicine research. It can be reached Monday through Friday, 8:30 a.m. to 5:00 p.m. Eastern time at (888) 644-6226 (voice and hearing impaired line). The address is NCCAM Clearinghouse, P.O. Box 8218, Silver Spring, MD 20907-8218. On-line it's found at http://nccam.nih.gov/nccam/clearinghouse/.

The Mayo Clinic

What can this renowned hospital do for you? Mainly, provide you with extensive health information about a variety of diseases through its Web site (www.mayohealth.org). There, you can look up information about medications, get current health information, or visit one of its "centers" for research on a specific condition or topic. For first-aid info, go right to www.mayohealth.org/mayo/library/htm/firstaid.htm for a library of choices.

As long as hospital Web sites are the topic, here's another: www.intelihealth.com. This relatively new site is backed by John Hopkins University and its health system and offers plenty of helpful information, including sites designed just for kids.

National Clearinghouse of Alcohol and Drug Information (NCADI)

The NCADI is an information service under the auspices of the U.S. Department of Health & Human Services. It's the world's largest resource for up-to-date information about drug and alcohol abuse, and it puts those resources at your fingertips through its Web site and information hot line. Over the phone, you can request brochures and fact sheets on alcohol, smoking, drugs, and related topics or inquire about intervention and treatment resources. And that's not all: On request, they'll do customized searches of their vast databases and deliver you the results.

To contact the NCADI, call (800) 662-4357; (800) 662-9832 (Spanish); (800) 228-0427 (hearing-impaired); or (301) 468-6433 (local). The organization's address is Box 2345, Rockville, MD 20847-2345. On-line it's found at www.health.org.

The Nemours Foundation and the American Medical Association

Together, these two groups have put together extensive on-line resources regarding children's health, providing particularly helpful information about safety and first aid. Their sister Web sites are www.kidshealth.org (which was put together with the help of the American Academy of Pediatrics, among other groups) and www.ama-assn.org/insight/h_focus/nemours. Look for information from everything about the stresses of parenting to what to put in your first-aid kit.

Want to write them? Here's the address: The Nemours Foundation Center for Children's Health Media, Alfred I. duPont Hospital for Children, 1600 Rockland Road, Wilmington, DE 19803; (302) 651-4046.

Index

• **C** •

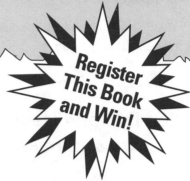

We want to hear from you!

Visit **http://my2cents.dummies.com** to register this book and tell us how you liked it!

✔ Get entered in our monthly prize giveaway.

✔ Give us feedback about this book — tell us what you like best, what you like least, or maybe what you'd like to ask the author and us to change!

✔ Let us know any other ...*For Dummies*® topics that interest you.

Your feedback helps us determine what books to publish, tells us what coverage to add as we revise our books, and lets us know whether we're meeting your needs as a ...*For Dummies* reader. You're our most valuable resource, and what you have to say is important to us!

Not on the Web yet? It's easy to get started with *Dummies 101*®: *The Internet For Windows*® *98* or *The Internet For Dummies*,® 6th Edition, at local retailers everywhere.

Or let us know what you think by sending us a letter at the following address:

...*For Dummies* Book Registration
Dummies Press
7260 Shadeland Station, Suite 100
Indianapolis, IN 46256-3917
Fax 317-596-5498

BESTSELLING
BOOK SERIES

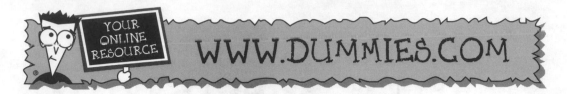

Discover Dummies Online!

The Dummies Web Site is your fun and friendly online resource for the latest information about *...For Dummies®* books and your favorite topics. The Web site is the place to communicate with us, exchange ideas with other *...For Dummies* readers, chat with authors, and have fun!

Ten Fun and Useful Things You Can Do at www.dummies.com

1. Win free *...For Dummies* books and more!
2. Register your book and be entered in a prize drawing.
3. Meet your favorite authors through the IDG Books Author Chat Series.
4. Exchange helpful information with other *...For Dummies* readers.
5. Discover other great *...For Dummies* books you must have!
6. Purchase Dummieswear™ exclusively from our Web site.
7. Buy *...For Dummies* books online.
8. Talk to us. Make comments, ask questions, get answers!
9. Download free software.
10. Find additional useful resources from authors.

Link directly to these ten fun and useful things at
http://www.dummies.com/10useful

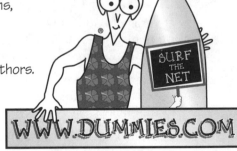

For other technology titles from IDG Books Worldwide, go to
www.idgbooks.com

Not on the Web yet? It's easy to get started with *Dummies 101®: The Internet For Windows®98* or *The Internet For Dummies®, 6th Edition,* at local retailers everywhere.

Find other *...For Dummies* books on these topics:
Business • Career • Databases • Food & Beverage • Games • Gardening • Graphics • Hardware
Health & Fitness • Internet and the World Wide Web • Networking • Office Suites
Operating Systems • Personal Finance • Pets • Programming • Recreation • Sports
Spreadsheets • Teacher Resources • Test Prep • Word Processing